ILEOSTOMY DIET

POST-SURGERY NUTRITION FOR OSTOMATE ABDOMINAL WELLNESS

Rapid Ileostomy Recovery Cookbook Solution On Beginners Recipes To Help Stoma, Reduce Swelling, Ease Digestion And Nourishment

DR. RUBEN BERRY

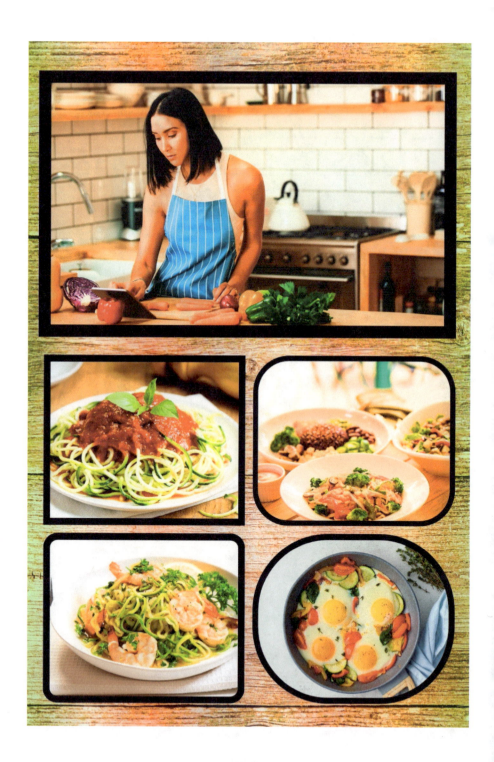

DISCLAIMER

This book's content is only meant to be used for general informative purposes. It is not intended to replace expert medical guidance, diagnosis, or care. When in doubt about a medical problem, never hesitate to consult your doctor or another trained healthcare professional.

This book's contents shouldn't be regarded as a replacement for medical advice. The food and lifestyle suggestions may not be appropriate for every person and are based on research and general understanding at the time of writing. For specific guidance, readers should speak with their healthcare practitioners.

Any particular person, product, website, organization, or other entity referenced in this book is not endorsed, recommended, or associated in any way by the author. The references are provided solely for informational purposes and do not indicate support.

It is advised that readers independently confirm the facts, particularly concerning dietary guidelines, medical problems, and product usage. Any direct or indirect effects arising from the use or use of the material included in this book are not to be held against the author or the publisher.

The author has taken every precaution to guarantee that the information in this book is correct as of the date of release. Nonetheless, the author disclaims all duty for any errors or omissions and does not guarantee the information's authenticity, dependability, or completeness.

You understand and accept the conditions of this disclaimer by reading this book. Please do not use this book if you disagree with these terms.

BRIEF DETAILS OD WHAT YOU WILL LEARN IN THIS BOOK

This invaluable guide, "Ileostomy Diet: Post Surgery Nutrition for Ostomate Abdominal Wellness," is a comprehensive resource that meticulously addresses the multifaceted aspects of life after ileostomy surgery. The first section dives deep into understanding the intricacies of ileostomy surgery, emphasizing the significance of adopting proper nutrition as a crucial component of the recovery process. This book uniquely merges practical advice with a positive mindset, fostering resilience and empowerment among ostomates.

Delving into the nutritional realm, the guide unveils an array of essential nutrients tailored specifically for ileostomy patients. By offering a detailed overview of key nutrients and emphasizing the importance of hydration, this book guides readers toward a customized nutrient intake that caters to their individual needs. The emphasis on hydration is particularly crucial, ensuring ostomates maintain optimal health and vitality.

A standout feature of this guide is its practical approach to building a balanced ileostomy diet. It expertly navigates the complexities of meal planning, incorporating nutrient-rich elements while providing insights into portion control and meal frequency. The section on safely integrating fiber showcases this book's commitment to offering not just information but actionable steps toward digestive well-being.

Navigating the culinary landscape becomes more manageable with the inclusion of foods to embrace and avoid. Readers gain insights into ostomy-friendly choices that ease digestion, along with tips on gradually introducing new foods. This book takes a holistic approach by addressing not just nutritional needs but also strategies to manage abdominal swelling and discomfort through gentle exercises.

The inclusion of quick and simple healing recipes elevates this guide to a practical cookbook solution. Nutrient-packed smoothies, healing soups, and easily digestible meals become essential tools in the recovery journey. Cooking techniques catered to ostomates, such as easy-to-digest methods and meal preparation tips, enhance the overall culinary experience, ensuring convenience without compromising nutrition.

Beyond the realm of nutrition, the guide extends its reach to address digestive challenges, providing practical tips on handling gas and odor issues. Lifestyle adjustments for improved digestion demonstrate a holistic approach to ostomy care. The emphasis on nourishing snack ideas and strategies for socializing and dining out contributes to a well-rounded guide that promotes sustained energy and confidence in various social settings.

Crucially, this book embraces the emotional and mental aspects of recovery. It guides readers through coping with body image changes, building a robust support system, and incorporating mindfulness and stress management techniques. The inclusion of topics like traveling with an ileostomy and long-term care ensures that readers are equipped not just for immediate recovery but for a fulfilling and empowered lifestyle.

BONUS: We have provided easy-to-follow 23 quick and simple healing recipes and preparatory procedures for ostomates' nutritional wellness, illustrated procedures you can easily implement which is believed to speed up your journey as you proceed with this book, your final bus stop.

In its totality, "Ileostomy Diet" transcends the conventional boundaries of post-surgery guides. It is an uplifting and engaging companion that empowers individuals on their journey to recovery, celebrating milestones, fostering resilience, and inspiring others to embrace a healthy and fulfilled lifestyle.

[13]

CHAPTER ONE

INTRODUCTION TO ILEOSTOMY

Understanding Ileostomy Surgery

Creating an artificial opening in the abdominal wall called a stoma, through which the small intestine is transported to the surface, is known as ileostomy surgery. When it becomes necessary to reroute the ileum—the lower portion of the small intestine—outside the body, this surgical procedure is usually carried out. Conditions including colon cancer, inflammatory bowel illness, or specific congenital defects may require this.

The process of digestion is profoundly changed when an ileostomy is created. Bowel habits are significantly altered as a result of the digestive tract's rerouting, which avoids the colon and eliminates digestive waste. Now that the patient's stool is being ejected through the stoma, it can be difficult for them to get used to this adjustment at first. Individuals who have an ileostomy must comprehend the alterations to their anatomy and how they will affect their day-to-day functioning.

Following ileostomy surgery, patients frequently experience a range of emotions, such as anxiety, dread, and future uncertainty. To assist people in adjusting to the psychological and physical implications of having an ileostomy, healthcare providers must offer thorough education and assistance throughout this time. Patient's quality of life is improved and their ability to actively participate in their treatment is increased when they have a thorough grasp of the procedure and its consequences.

Following Surgery, Adequate Nutrition Is Crucial

Maintaining a healthy, balanced diet is crucial for those recovering from ileostomy surgery to improve their general well-being. Because of the potential impact of the changed digestive process on nutritional absorption, food choices must be carefully considered. The goals of a carefully thought-out ileostomy diet are to manage potential problems, avoid dehydration, and replace vital nutrients.

Dehydration from increased fluid loss through the stoma is one of the main problems after ileostomy surgery. It is essential to consume enough fluids, such as water and electrolyte-rich drinks, to reduce this risk. Incorporating a range of nutrient-dense meals is also crucial to guaranteeing that people obtain a wide range of vitamins and minerals. These foods include fruits, vegetables, lean meats, and whole grains.

Consuming too much or too little fiber can affect transit time and stool consistency, so it's important to carefully check your intake. To ensure that dietary advice is customized to each person's needs and tastes, speaking with a healthcare provider or registered dietitian is essential. Dietary modifications will be guided by weight, energy, and general digestive health monitoring, supporting appropriate nutrition and reducing the risk of problems following ileostomy surgery.

Embracing a Positive Mindset

For those who have an ileostomy, emotional health is crucial to their overall adjustment and recuperation process. Navigating the obstacles that may appear during the post-surgery period requires adopting an optimistic outlook. People may see having an ileostomy as a positive step toward a higher quality of life if they are aware that it is a life-saving procedure and a tool for enhancing health.

Loved ones, support groups, and medical experts can all make a big difference in helping to cultivate a positive outlook. Promoting candid dialogue about worries, anxieties, and changes can assist people in managing their feelings and taking charge of their circumstances. Recognizing the psychological effects of the surgery and offering services for mental health treatment are essential.

Including activities that encourage calmness, awareness, and stress relief can also help foster a good outlook. Emotional well-being requires hobbies, social interaction, and preserving a feeling of normalcy in day-to-day living. People with ileostomies can develop resilience, adaptability, and a positive view on their road toward abdominal wholeness by actively addressing the emotional aspects of their condition.

CHAPTER TWO

ESSENTIAL NUTRIENTS FOR OSTOMATES

Overview of Key Nutrients for Ileostomy Patients

It is imperative for persons who have had ileostomy surgery to maintain appropriate nutrition. Following this surgery, there are notable changes in the digestive tract that impact the absorption of nutrients and the process of digestion. Ileostomates must thus monitor their diet carefully to make sure they get the vital elements for good general health and well-being.

Electrolyte homeostasis is a major concern for people with ileostomies. The small intestine is rerouted during the procedure, which has an impact on the absorption of electrolytes like sodium, potassium, and chloride. If not appropriately handled, this change may result in electrolyte imbalances and dehydration. It is essential to consume enough of these electrolytes to avoid problems and preserve regular body processes.

Another essential component for ileostomates is protein, which is vital for both general bodily function and tissue repair. Patients must eat high-quality protein sources because the surgical treatment may have an impact on how well they absorb protein. Dairy products, eggs, plant-based proteins, and lean meats can all help satisfy protein requirements and promote the healing process.

Minerals and vitamins are necessary for many physiological functions, and ileostomates require special attention to certain micronutrients. For example, abnormalities in the gastrointestinal tract may result in a deficiency of vitamin B12. Sufficient consumption of B12 via supplements or meals fortified with iron is required to avoid B12 deficiency and associated health problems.

To support regular bowel movements and aid in digestion, fiber is an essential part of a healthy diet. Ileostomy patients must use caution while consuming large amounts of fiber, as this may cause discomfort or obstructions. It's best to add fiber gradually and keep an eye on how it affects bowel movements.

In conclusion, individuals with ileostomies need to concentrate on eating a balanced diet that meets their specific dietary requirements. Sufficient consumption of vitamins, minerals, protein, and electrolytes is necessary to support general health, encourage healing, and avoid difficulties.

Tailoring Nutrition Consumption for Patients with Ileostomies

For ileostomy patients, a key component of a post-surgery diet is individualized nutrient intake. A careful and individualized strategy is necessary to guarantee that each person receives the proper mix of nutrients for maximum health and well-being because of the distinctive changes in the digestive system.

Modifying meal frequencies and portion sizes is an important factor to take into account. Smaller, more frequent meals spread out throughout the day may aid in improved nutrient absorption and digestion for ileostomy patients. Additionally, by avoiding overtaxing the digestive system, this method can lower the chance of pain or difficulties.

For ileostomates, electrolyte levels must be regularly monitored and adjusted. It is crucial to collaborate closely with medical personnel to ascertain the proper intake of sodium, potassium, and chloride because the surgery modifies the body's ability to absorb electrolytes. Frequent blood testing can assist in determining electrolyte levels and help direct dietary or supplement changes that may be required.

When it comes to dietary intake customization for ileostomy patients, protein needs to be the main focus. A sufficient and varied amino acid profile can be achieved by including a range of protein sources, including lean meats, fish, eggs, dairy, and plant-based foods. To satisfy specific needs, protein supplements may also be taken into consideration with the advice of medical professionals.

It is equally important to customize vitamin and mineral consumption. Blood level monitoring regularly can help determine when to supplement with certain minerals, like calcium, iron, and vitamin B12. Including a range of foods high in nutrients in the diet can help create a well-rounded nutritional profile.

Furthermore, patients with ileostomies must modify their fiber intake. Although fiber is typically beneficial to digestive health, ileostomy patients must find a balance. To avoid issues like blockages, soluble fiber should be gradually added and its impact on bowel function should be monitored.

In conclusion, an individualized and adaptable strategy is needed to customize dietary intake for ileostomy patients. To effectively ensure that dietary requirements are satisfied, promoting recovery and long-term well-being, collaboration with healthcare professionals, regular monitoring, and changes based on individual needs are essential.

Tips for Hydration for Ostomates

For ostomates, especially those who have had ileostomy surgery, maintaining adequate water is essential to good health. Maintaining general health, avoiding problems, and assisting the body's healing processes all depend heavily on hydration. Ostomates must thus take extra care to monitor their fluid intake and develop plans for staying properly hydrated.

Hydration is even more important for ileostomy patients since their changed digestive systems can result in higher fluid loss. Osteomates are more susceptible to dehydration because of variations in the digestive tract's ability to absorb water. It's crucial to drink enough water throughout the day to help fight this.

For ostomates, incorporating electrolyte-rich beverages into their regular regimen is a beneficial hydration approach. Electrolytes, like potassium and sodium, are essential for preserving the body's fluid balance. Sports drinks, homemade electrolyte solutions, or coconut water can all be consumed to help replace these vital minerals and keep dehydration at bay.

For ostomates, observing the color of their urine is a straightforward but effective way to gauge their level of hydration. While dark yellow or amber may indicate dehydration, a light, pale yellow tint indicates appropriate hydration. To guarantee appropriate hydration, ostomates should strive for a pale yellow tint in their urine.

Spreading out your daily fluid intake evenly is another ostomate hydration strategy. Drinking water or other hydrating drinks regularly might help the body absorb fluids more efficiently and avoid overloading the digestive system. For ileostomy patients in particular, this strategy is crucial since large amounts of fluids ingested at once may transit through the digestive tract too fast, increasing fluid loss.

Apart from drinks, including items that are high in moisture in the diet can also help increase the amount of fluid consumed overall. High-water fruits and vegetables, like oranges, cucumbers, and watermelon, can be a great way to increase hydration.

Ostomates must learn to listen to their body and act quickly if they exhibit symptoms of dehydration. It is important to pay attention to symptoms such as increased thirst, dark urine, dry mouth, and dizziness. It is imperative to consult a physician and modify fluid consumption to avoid issues linked to dehydration.

In conclusion, for ostomates—especially those who have an ileostomy—staying properly hydrated is an essential part of their post-surgery nutrition.

By following these hydration recommendations—which include keeping an eye on the color of urine, ingesting electrolyte-rich drinks, distributing their fluid intake, and including foods high in water content—ostomates can maintain optimal levels of hydration for better health and well-being.

CHAPTER THREE

BUILDING A BALANCED ILEOSTOMY DIET

Designing a Nutrient-Rich Meal Plan for Ileostomy Patients:

For those who have an ileostomy, creating a meal plan that is both balanced and nutrient-rich is essential since they must manage their specific dietary needs and make sure they get enough nutrients. It's critical to concentrate on a diet that supports general well-being, gives energy, and aids in recovery following surgery. To satisfy the body's nutritional demands, a range of nutrient-dense foods must be included.

A key component of a nutrient-dense ileostomy diet includes a wide variety of food groups. This guarantees a wide range of vital vitamins and minerals to support the body's functioning and help in the healing process. Lean protein sources including fish, fowl, and tofu can aid in the preservation and regeneration of tissue. Consuming a range of vibrant fruits and vegetables contributes fiber, vitamins, and antioxidants that support digestive health in general. Complex carbs and whole grains are necessary for maintaining energy levels and enhancing the patient's general health and vigor.

Maintaining adequate hydration is similarly crucial for ileostomy patients. Drinking enough water promotes healthy digestion, guards against problems, and helps keep electrolyte balance. Patients should make sure they drink enough water throughout the day and include items high in water, such as fruits and vegetables, in their diet. It's important to keep an eye on your hydration levels, especially since ileostomy patients are more likely to become dehydrated because of their altered digestive processes.

It can be helpful to take into account the consistency of the foods in addition to concentrating on particular dietary groups. Patients with ileostomies may find it beneficial to start with softer, more easily digested foods and then progressively introduce a greater variety of textures as their digestive systems adjust. To tailor the meal plan to each person's needs, including age, weight, and any underlying medical concerns, it is important to collaborate closely with a qualified dietitian or healthcare expert.

Meal Frequency and Portion Control for Patients with Ileostomies:

For those who have an ileostomy, careful meal frequency and effective portion control are essential to their overall health. Following surgery, the digestive process is altered, thus controlling meal sizes helps avoid overloading the digestive system and reduces the chance of complications.

For ileostomy patients, breaking up meals into smaller, more frequent portions throughout the day is frequently advised. This method helps avoid overburdening the digestive tract in addition to facilitating simpler digestion. Meals that are smaller and more frequent can help improve nutritional absorption and ease the burden on the digestive system. Patients must learn to listen to their bodies, identify fullness cues, and modify portion amounts accordingly.

Another important component of portion control for ileostomy patients is balancing macronutrients. Every meal should have a combination of carbohydrates, proteins, and fats to fulfill total nutritional demands and assist deliver sustained energy. It is imperative to customize the macronutrient distribution to each patient's tolerance and desire, though, as some may have more difficulty breaking down particular food groups.

Optimizing meal timing throughout the day can also help with improved absorption and digestion. Smaller meals spread evenly throughout the day are found by many ileostomy patients to help manage symptoms and increase comfort. Large meals should be avoided, especially right before bed, as this might help to reduce discomfort and other potential problems while you sleep.

Including Fiber in Ileostomy Patients in a Safe Way:

It takes careful planning and consideration to include fiber in an ileostomy patient's diet without endangering the health of their stoma. Ileostomy patients may need to modify their intake of fiber, even though it's essential for maintaining digestive health overall, to avoid difficulties.

Patients with ileostomies typically tolerate soluble fiber better, which can be found in foods like potatoes, bananas, and oats. It turns into a gel-like substance when dissolved in water, which may be easier on the digestive tract. Conversely, some people may find it more difficult to tolerate insoluble fiber, which is present in whole grains and some vegetables. Patients must try a variety of fiber sources and types to determine what is most effective for them.

For ileostomy patients, including fiber in the diet, gradually is essential. By starting small and progressively increasing over time, the danger of pain or difficulties is reduced and the digestive system is given time to adjust. A certified dietitian or other healthcare professional can offer individualized advice on the right kind and quantity of fiber for each person, taking into consideration tolerance levels and unique medical problems.

Assessing stoma output and noticing any variations in consistency might assist patients in determining how much fiber they can tolerate. When consuming more fiber, it's important to drink enough water because fiber absorbs water and can make stools bulkier. Consuming enough fluids promotes the digestive system's healthy operation and aids in the prevention of issues like obstructions.

To sum up, planning a healthy ileostomy diet requires paying close attention to foods high in nutrients, controlling portion sizes, and introducing fiber gradually. Developing a customized diet plan in close collaboration with healthcare providers promotes overall abdominal well-being and aids in the healing process following surgery.

CHAPTER FOUR

FOODS TO EMBRACE AND AVOID

Ostomy-Friendly Foods for Easy Digestion:

Following ileostomy surgery, a seamless transition necessitates the adoption of an ostomy-friendly diet that facilitates easy digestion and fosters gut well-being. Ostomates—people who have had ileostomy surgery—can benefit from relief and comfort when they include particular items in their daily diet.

A diet that is ostomy-friendly must prioritize items that are easy to digest. Choosing soft and cooked veggies like spinach, zucchini, and carrots will help your digestion go more smoothly.

These veggies give the body the nutrition it needs without overtaxing the digestive system. Lean protein sources, like skinless chicken, fish, and tofu, help to guarantee a balanced diet while reducing the chance of stomach distress.

Soft fruits that are easy on the digestive system, such as cooked apples, ripe avocados, and bananas, are great options for ostomates. These fruits don't irritate the skin and offer vital vitamins and minerals. Furthermore, eating refined carbohydrates in moderation—such as white rice and pasta—can help maintain a well-rounded diet that facilitates simple digestion.

For ostomates, dairy items can be a challenging area because some people may develop lactose sensitivity after surgery. Choosing lactose-free substitutes, such as yogurt or almond milk, may be an appropriate remedy. Incorporating foods high in probiotics, such as yogurt with live cultures, can also support a gut environment that is healthy and facilitates digestion.

Ostomy sufferers must stay hydrated. Maintaining a well-lubricated digestive system and preventing dehydration are two benefits of drinking lots of water. Drinking water frequently during the day, particularly in between meals, can help maintain ideal hydration levels without pushing too much fluid out of the stoma.

To summarize, ostomates can greatly benefit from an ostomy-friendly diet that emphasizes readily digestible meals, lean meats, soft fruits, and cautious dairy selections. This can also help to ensure that ostomates have a favorable post-surgery nutritional experience.

Foods that Could Be Upsetting or Blocking:

Ostomates must use caution when navigating the post-ileostomy terrain because some meals can cause discomfort or obstructions. Although eating a balanced diet is important, eliminating some foods can help to avoid issues and promote a quicker recovery.

High-fiber foods are one area to go cautiously. Even though fiber is generally seen as healthful, ostomates may need to start with a lower intake. Foods that can be difficult to digest and may cause blockages include raw vegetables, nuts, and seeds. The digestive system can gradually adjust by introducing these high-fiber foods in lesser amounts over time.

Some fruits, such as citrus fruits and berries with seeds, can be difficult for ostomates to consume. The small seeds and hard membranes may cause discomfort or obstructions. Choosing seedless and peeled types or eating these fruits in moderation can help reduce the risk.

Even though they are high in nutrients, whole grains might cause issues for ostomates. Certain foods, such as quinoa, brown rice, and whole wheat bread, might irritate the stomach or clog it. It may be safer to start with refined grains and gradually add whole grains back in moderation.

Tough or stringy meats may be difficult for the digestive system to process, which could be uncomfortable. Choosing soft meats and making sure you chew well before swallowing can help avoid stomach problems.

Regarding dairy products, some ostomates may develop lactose intolerance after surgery. It can be necessary to switch out lactose-containing dairy products, like whole milk and some cheeses, with lactose-free ones to prevent stomach pain.

It is important to be aware of personal sensitivities. Certain ostomates may experience discomfort from spicy foods, fizzy drinks, and high caffeine intake. Maintaining abdominal wellness requires keeping an eye on how the body reacts to these things and adjusting as necessary.

In conclusion, ostomates can prevent discomfort and blockages and have a more favorable post-surgery experience by being aware of the potential dangers of specific meals and exercising caution when consuming high-fiber, difficult, or possibly irritating products.

Advice for Introducing New Foods Gradually:

After ileostomy surgery, the road to regaining a varied and fulfilling diet entails introducing new foods gradually and thoughtfully. Ostomates can gain from a methodical approach that takes into account the flexibility of their digestive system, guaranteeing a seamless transition and fostering intestinal health.

Starting with foods that are easily digested is a basic suggestion. It can be easier to adjust by selecting foods that are well-cooked and have a softer texture, as the digestive system may be more sensitive at first. When starting to reintroduce solid foods, steamed veggies, soft meats, and cooked fruits are great options.

When it comes to increasing the range of foods in an ostomy-friendly diet, it's best to go slowly but steadily. Ostomates should concentrate on one food item at a time rather than introducing several new foods at once. This facilitates the identification of any potential triggers or sensitivities by providing a clear picture of how the body responds to each new addition.

Food journals might be an invaluable resource for you at this time. A thorough summary can be obtained by keeping track of the kinds of meals eaten, the portions taken, and any symptoms or responses that may arise. This notebook can be used to spot trends and make well-informed choices about the foods you should include or stay away from in the future.

Portion control is very important, especially when introducing new meals that may irritate the digestive system or have a higher fiber content. The digestive system can adjust to larger amounts over time by starting with smaller ones and gradually increasing them.

A well-balanced diet is guaranteed when a range of food groups are included. To find a combination that works for their unique tolerances and tastes, osteomates can experiment with different kinds of fats, carbs, and proteins. This method not only enhances nutritional diversity but also improves the post-operative diet's palatability.

Finally, seeking advice from a medical professional or a qualified dietitian with expertise in ostomy nutrition might offer tailored recommendations. These experts may provide customized guidance based on a person's unique nutritional needs, medical history, and current state of health.

In conclusion, a methodical and patient approach is required when introducing new foods gradually after ileostomy. Keeping a food log, introducing one food at a time, concentrating on readily digested foods, paying attention to portion sizes, and getting professional advice are all helpful steps in the direction of a varied and well-balanced diet for ostomates.

CHAPTER FIVE

MANAGING SWELLING AND DISCOMFORT

Strategies to Reduce Abdominal Swelling

Concerns about abdominal swelling are frequent among those who have had ileostomy surgery. Although some degree of swelling is expected during the recovery phase, it is critical to appropriately manage it for the optimal health of ostomates. Focusing on a customized and well-balanced diet is one important tactic. Eating more often and in smaller portions can reduce bloating and avoid overtaxing the digestive system. Ostomates should chew their meals well and stay away from items that cause gas, like carbonated drinks and some vegetables like beans and cabbage, as they might cause distension in the abdomen.

Reducing stomach swelling requires adequate hydration. Ostomates should continue to consume enough fluids to avoid dehydration, which can make swelling worse.

But it's important to pay attention to the kinds of liquids you drink.

Carbonated beverages have the potential to cause pain by introducing extra gas into the digestive tract. It can be advantageous to choose water, herbal teas, and other non-carbonated drinks.

Probiotics may also help to maintain a healthier digestive tract when added to the diet. Yogurt and other fermented foods include probiotics, which encourage the growth of good bacteria in the gut to help with digestion and may lessen bloating. Ostomates should speak with their doctors before starting any new supplements or making significant dietary adjustments.

Using the proper ostomy pouching system is crucial to reducing belly swelling, in addition to nutritional considerations. Leaks and pain can be avoided, lowering the possibility of skin irritation and inflammation, by making sure the pouch fits properly and replacing it regularly. Speak with a stoma care nurse or other medical expert for advice on which pouching system is best for your needs. This will help you choose more comfortably around your abdomen.

Easy Exercises for Patients with Ileostomies

For ileostomy patients, adding mild workouts to the regimen can be a helpful way to control abdominal edema. As the body takes some time to heal after surgery, it's important to begin with low-impact exercises. Walking is a great option because it helps to prevent problems like blood clots and increases blood circulation.

Exercises that strengthen the core can be very helpful for people who have ileostomies. These exercises, which include mild abdominal contractions and pelvic tilts, serve to increase abdominal muscle tone, supporting the stoma and lowering the risk of hernias. But it's important to take your time with these workouts and stay away from intense activities that can strain your abdominal muscles.

Stretching routines and yoga can also be quite effective in fostering relaxation and flexibility. Engaging in these activities improves mental and emotional health in addition to physical well-being. Including deep breathing techniques in your routine can help you relax even more, which will lessen stress and any discomfort that may arise from swelling in your abdomen.

Ileostomy patients need to speak with their healthcare providers before starting any fitness program. Experts can offer tailored advice depending on a patient's unique medical circumstances and the particulars of the ileostomy procedure. For ostomates to exercise safely and effectively, a regimen that gradually increases intensity after brief, manageable sessions is essential.

Keeping an eye on and resolving discomfort

Proactive monitoring and prompt intervention are necessary for the effective management of discomfort following ileostomy surgery. To spot any indications of irritation, inflammation, or infection, the stoma and peristomal skin must be regularly inspected. Ostomates should be aware of any changes in the stoma's color, size, or output as these may be signs of serious problems that need to be checked out by a doctor.

To alleviate discomfort, it is essential to closely monitor dietary practices. Ostomates who are tracking the effects of various foods on their digestive tract should maintain a food journal. By recognizing your trigger foods and modifying your diet appropriately, you can greatly reduce your suffering. Furthermore, seeking advice from a licensed dietitian or nutritionist can offer individualized recommendations for tailoring the diet to promote belly wellbeing.

It is essential to have proactive communication with medical specialists to swiftly address any emergent concerns. Ostomates ought to feel comfortable talking about any discomfort, bowel changes, or mental difficulties they may be going through. Healthcare professionals can provide individualized treatments, such as prescription modifications, nutritional advice, or connections to specialized support services.

In summary, ileostomy patients must take a multifaceted approach that includes careful monitoring, mild activity, and dietary modifications to effectively manage swelling and discomfort. By implementing these techniques in conjunction with medical specialists, ostomates can better their overall quality of life and improve their abdominal well-being.

CHAPTER SIX

QUICK AND SIMPLE HEALING RECIPES

Nutrient-Packed Smoothies and Juices

Smoothies and drinks that are high in nutrients are an integral part of the ileostomy diet, providing a delightful and easy method to replace vital nutrients and support abdominal well-being following surgery. These drinks support the healing process by offering a concentrated dosage of vitamins, minerals, and water.

Think about adding items like leafy greens, fresh fruits, and protein-rich sources like plant-based protein powder or yogurt to make a restorative smoothie. Antioxidant-rich berries can help lower inflammation, while fruits and vegetables' high fiber content promotes healthy digestive systems. A dash of almond milk or coconut water improves flavor and guarantees adequate hydration, which is necessary to preserve electrolyte balance.

Juices can be just as helpful since they provide vital nutrients in a liquid form. Freshly squeezed fruits and vegetables are a better choice because they are packed with antioxidants and digestive enzymes that promote overall health. For example, carrot and ginger juice may have anti-inflammatory properties and aid in digestive tract stability. Try different combinations of tastes to find ones that maximize nutritional advantages and fit your taste preferences.

It is noteworthy that persons who have an ileostomy may need to exercise caution when it comes to high-fiber substances, as too much fiber may cause discomfort. A delicate but efficient approach to post-surgery nourishment is ensured by customizing smoothies and liquids to individual tolerances.

Nutrient-dense smoothies and juices are a great way for people to satisfy their nutritional needs without stressing out their digestive systems, and they also help in the healing process.

Remedy Broths & Soups

The foundation of the ileostomy diet is healing soups and broths, which provide support, nutrition, and simple digestion for those recovering from surgery and working toward gut health. These comforting and warm mixtures offer a gentle means of introducing vital nutrients and fostering healing.

Particularly bone broth is well known for its therapeutic qualities. Bone broth, rich in collagen, amino acids, and minerals, promotes digestive health, lowers inflammation, and facilitates tissue healing. It offers a supply of nutrients that are readily absorbed, which is essential for ileostomy patients while they adjust to altered digestive processes.

Soups made from vegetables, like a straightforward carrot and potato soup or a comforting butternut squash soup, are a great way to receive enough vitamins and minerals without overtaxing the digestive system. To make these soups smoother and simpler to stomach and absorb nutrients from, you can mix them.

It's important to steer clear of overusing high-fiber elements in healing soups, as these might be difficult for the digestive system to process. Rather, concentrate on adding simple-to-digest veggies, lean meats, and low-residue grains to offer a nutrient-dense, yet gentle, alternative for nourishment following surgery.

Including therapeutic soups and broths in the ileostomy, the diet promotes both physical healing and a feeling of comfort and sustenance while the body heals.

Comfortable and Simple to Digest Meals

Meals that are soft and easily absorbed are essential to an ileostomy diet because they provide a balance between nutrition and comfort for those recovering from abdominal surgery. These dishes emphasize using mild ingredients that are easy on the stomach while yet making sure that important nutrients are consumed.

Select tender, well-cooked veggies such as steamed spinach, zucchini, or carrots. These veggies facilitate easier digestion by offering vitamins and minerals without the added strain of a high fiber content. Sweet potatoes or mashed potatoes are great options because they are easy on the stomach and provide a decent amount of energy and important nutrients.

Soft meals with protein sources, such as fish, tofu, or baked or poached chicken, can aid in general healing and muscle restoration. To make proteins easier for the digestive system to digest, make sure they are prepared while they are still delicate.

When cooked properly, grains like quinoa and white rice can be included in soft, easily digested meals and serve as a source of carbs for long-lasting energy. Foods that are highly seasoned or processed should be avoided because they can irritate the digestive system.

Post-surgery feeding can be made easier for those with an ileostomy by emphasizing soft, readily digestible meals. These meals not only aid in the physical healing process but also facilitate a more seamless shift to a reduced diet, thereby enhancing abdominal well-being.

CHAPTER SEVEN

COOKING TECHNIQUES FOR OSTOMATES

Easy-to-Digest Cooking Methods

It becomes crucial to prioritize easy-to-digest cooking techniques when creating a diet for someone who has an ileostomy. The digestive system changes significantly following surgery, and some cooking methods can assist reduce stress on the gastrointestinal tract while maintaining adequate food absorption.

For ostomates, steaming is a fantastic cooking technique. The limited use of oils or fats facilitates simpler digestion while maintaining the natural flavors and nutrients in food. Seared to perfection, vegetables, fish, and chicken make a delicious and easily digestible option for individuals adjusting to an ileostomy diet. Boiling is also an appropriate method because it tenderizes food without requiring a lot of fat.

For ileostomates, slow cooking emerges as a practical and comforting option. This technique produces soft, readily digested meals by cooking food over low heat for an extended amount of time. Slow-cooked stews, soups, and casseroles offer a variety of flavors without sacrificing nutritional content. The longer cooking time helps people with altered digestive systems digest meats and vegetables more easily since it breaks down the fibers.

When executed precisely, grilling can also be a culinary technique that is beneficial for ileostomies. It adds a smokey flavor without using a lot of fats or oils. Grilling lean foods, such as chicken or fish, results in a delicious texture that doesn't burden the digestive system. Foods that have been marinated before grilling have better flavor and are more tender, which is better for the digestive system.

When it comes to lipids in cooking, using healthier substitutes like olive oil might facilitate simpler digestion. Cooking with monounsaturated fats preserves the harmony between taste and dietary requirements. Minimal oil stir-frying facilitates rapid cooking without sacrificing the entire digestive experience. Achieving a balanced intake of essential nutrients without overburdening the digestive system is crucial.

In conclusion, choosing cooking techniques that are simple to digest is crucial for people following an ileostomy diet. Cooking techniques such as steaming, boiling, slow cooking, and careful grilling can all be very important in making sure that meals are not only nourishing but also easy on the digestive system, encouraging ostomates' abdominal well-being.

Getting Meals Ready Ahead

Effective meal preparation is essential for ostomates to overcome the difficulties associated with an ileostomy diet. Making meals ahead of time not only expedites the cooking process but also guarantees a steady and nutritionally sound diet, which helps to maintain abdominal well-being after surgery.

When it comes to meal preparation for ileostomates, batch cooking shines. Setting aside time specifically to prepare bigger amounts of food enables people to prepare meals for the coming week. This approach lowers the risk of boredom by encouraging variation in the diet while also saving time. The basis for preparing a variety of wholesome meals is laid by bulk-preparing essentials like whole grains, lean proteins, and easily digested veggies.

Purchasing high-quality storage containers is an essential part of meal planning ahead of time. Using airtight containers reduces the chance of bacterial infection and helps keep food fresher longer. Meal portioning into smaller containers also makes reheating easier and guarantees that the flavor and nutritional value of each serving are maintained. This technique helps with portion control, which is important for keeping a balanced diet, in addition to being convenient.

For ileostomates, making a weekly meal plan is a smart move. This entails planning each day's meals while taking dietary requirements and preferences into account. In addition to encouraging a balanced diet, a well-thought-out plan relieves the burden of everyday meal planning. It gives people the freedom to concentrate on finding premium, ileostomy-friendly ingredients and guarantees they have everything they need to prepare healthy meals.

Meal preparation gains versatility when it incorporates items that are interchangeable and can be utilized in many recipes. A pot of quinoa or some roasted veggies, for example, might be the foundation for several meals during the week. This flexibility boosts productivity and gives you a creative outlet to make a variety of tasty dishes.

To sum up, planning meals ahead of time is essential to effective nutritional control for ileostomates. Incorporating adaptable ingredients, meal planning every week, batch cooking, and using high-quality storage solutions all help to create a smooth and nutrient-dense post-surgery diet strategy that promotes abdominal well-being.

Kitchen Appliances for Practicality

Using well-selected kitchen appliances can greatly simplify navigating the culinary scene as an ostomate. For those getting used to an ileostomy diet, these gadgets make meal preparation easier and more pleasurable by streamlining the cooking process and improving convenience.

For ileostomates, a high-quality blender is a multipurpose kitchen tool that can transform everything. There are so many things you can do with a blender, from making smoothies with easily digested fruits to making soups with finely mashed vegetables. Its capacity to reduce food into a smooth consistency guarantees that people can eat a wide range of meals high in nutrients without sacrificing their texture or digestion.

Purchasing a food processor gives roommates new opportunities in the kitchen. This device is great at dicing, slicing, and chopping food, saving labor-intensive manual labor. A food processor becomes a vital ally for people who are physically or mentally exhausted, as it makes it easier for them to prepare a wide variety of components for meals.

Slow cookers are a godsend for ileostomates looking for convenience because of their set-it-and-forget-it nature. With the help of these appliances, filling stews, soups, and casseroles can be made without continual supervision. Foods are made tender and easily digestible by the slow cooking method, which promotes stomach well-being without sacrificing flavor.

For people who value steaming in their cooking routine, an electric steamer becomes their go-to appliance. This appliance streamlines the steaming procedure, rendering it a hassle-free choice for cooking fish, poultry, and vegetables. Ileostomates require a delicate cooking procedure that preserves nutritional content, and this is provided by the regulated steam environment.

An air fryer is a useful addition to the kitchen toolkit for accurate cooking without using excessive amounts of fat. This appliance cooks food by using hot air to create a crispy outside without the need for deep frying. It makes it possible for people to savor the taste and texture of fried food in a way that is more palatable to their digestive systems.

In conclusion, ileostomates can greatly improve their cooking experience by choosing the appropriate kitchen appliances. A food processor, air fryer, blender, slow cooker, electric steamer, and slow cooker all provide unique contributions to convenience, providing effective meal prep options that maintain abdominal health for those following an ileostomy diet.

CHAPTER EIGHT

HANDLING DIGESTIVE CHALLENGES

Dealing with Gas and Odor Issues:

Managing the gas and odor problems that come with having an ileostomy is one of the main obstacles that ostomates have after surgery. People can adjust to their new normal more easily if they realize that this is a typical part of the digestive process. Gas cannot be eliminated, but there are ways to lessen its effects on day-to-day living.

The diet is a major factor in gas generation. Some foods can cause more gas, including beans, cabbage, and carbonated drinks. Ostomates ought to think about following a low-residue diet that restricts their intake of foods heavy in fiber and gas. To further minimize gas formation, chew food well and refrain from chatting while eating to minimize the quantity of air swallowed.

Selecting the appropriate pouching system is crucial for managing smells. These days, ostomy pouches are frequently furnished with filters that neutralize gas, offering comfort and discretion. Regularly emptying the pouch can also aid in avoiding the accumulation of odors. Ostomates should practice good hygiene and use deodorizing sprays or pouch liners as appropriate.

Accepting lifestyle adjustments can help ease gas and odor issues even more. Gas accumulation is lessened by physical activity, which also supports a healthy digestive system. Deep breathing and yoga are two relaxation practices that can help reduce the negative effects of stress on the digestive system. To retain discretion and confidence in social circumstances, it may be beneficial for ostomates to plan pouch changes at private moments.

Suggestions for Enhancing Satiety in the Stomach:

Following ileostomy surgery, achieving digestive comfort requires a combination of food decisions, hydration, and mindful eating practices. To find trigger foods and prevent discomfort, reintroducing foods into the diet gradually is essential.

Eating a healthy diet is dependent on staying hydrated. Ostomates should make it a point to stay hydrated throughout the day because dehydration might result in thicker excrement and possible obstructions. To avoid diluting digestive enzymes, it is better to sip water in between meals as opposed to eating big amounts during meals.

Yogurt and pills include probiotics, which can help with digestion and support a healthy gut flora. It's crucial to introduce them gradually, though, as some people could react negatively to shifts in the bacterial balance. To encourage regular bowel movements without creating obstructions, ostomates should focus on soluble fiber sources like rice, bananas, and oats when monitoring their fiber consumption.

Because eating smaller, more frequent meals eases the strain on the digestive tract, it can improve comfort with digestion. Eating with full teeth facilitates digestion and reduces gas in the stomach. Maintaining a food journal can help you spot trends and make well-informed dietary selections that support your digestive system's general health.

Modifications to Lifestyle to Improve Digestion:

After ileostomy surgery, maintaining optimal digestive health necessitates a comprehensive strategy that goes beyond food considerations. For ostomates, changing their way of life is essential to supporting improved digestion and general abdominal wellness.

Exercise regularly is essential for maintaining good digestion. In addition to encouraging bowel movements and lowering the risk of constipation, physical activity also aids in maintaining a healthy weight. To enhance general well-being, osteomates should partake in enjoyable activities like swimming, walking, or gentle aerobics.

Since stress can impair digestive function, stress management is crucial. Stress can be lessened by incorporating relaxation techniques like deep breathing exercises, mindfulness exercises, or meditation. Getting enough sleep is crucial since not getting enough sleep can interfere with digestion and make you feel uncomfortable all around.

For ostomates, establishing a schedule for meals and pouch changes might help make life more predictable. Better digestive health and the regulation of bowel motions are facilitated by mealtime and pouch management consistency. Anxiety can also be reduced by making advance plans for social gatherings and travel, which also guarantees that lodging and other necessities will be easily accessible.

In summary, a proactive strategy for controlling digestive issues following ileostomy surgery combines dietary decisions, lifestyle modifications, and an optimistic outlook. Ostomates can improve their overall abdominal well-being and digestive comfort by implementing these tips into their daily lives.

CHAPTER NINE

NOURISHING SNACK IDEAS

Portable and Easy-to-Carry Snacks:

Following ileostomy surgery, people must maintain a balanced diet to guarantee they get the nutrients they need and to support abdominal wellbeing. Snack selection is one area that needs careful thought, especially when it comes to lightweight and carrying snacks. This becomes particularly crucial for those who have an ileostomy since they must watch what they eat to avoid any issues.

Convenience is paramount when it comes to portable food. Choosing portable solutions can have a big impact on an ostomate's day-to-day activities. For example, nuts and seeds are small and densely packed with vital nutrients. Nuts like walnuts, pumpkin seeds, and almonds are good sources of fiber, protein, and omega-3 fatty acids. Their small size allows them to easily slip into a pocket or bag, making them the ideal snack for on-the-go.

Fresh fruit is also a great option for a portable snack. In addition to being nutrient-dense, apples, bananas, and grapes are also portable and don't require complex packaging. Slicing apples and serving them with almond butter or a tiny container of yogurt can improve the nutritious content of the snack while still making it convenient to eat anywhere. Dried fruits, like raisins or apricots, can be stored in a tiny container for a quick and energizing treat for people with a sweet craving.

In addition, the market provides a range of prepackaged, portion-controlled snacks designed to meet the needs of people who lead busy lives. Wholegrain crackers, cheese sticks, and individually wrapped nut bars are a few examples of them. With a well-balanced mix of fats, proteins, and carbohydrates, these snacks guarantee sustained energy without requiring a lot of planning or preparation.

Snacks that are lightweight and portable should be a part of an ileostomy diet because they promote general health and convenience. People can minimize any possible digestive system problems and maintain a healthy balance by selecting nutrient-dense foods.

Snacking Techniques for Long-Term Energy:

Developing smart snacking habits is essential for people adjusting to life after ileostomy surgery to maintain their energy levels all day. In addition to promoting general health, a healthy diet helps avert potential ileostomy-related problems. It's critical to concentrate on a variety of macronutrients, such as carbohydrates, proteins, and fats when snacking for sustained energy to give a consistent release of energy.

Incorporating complex carbohydrates into snacks is one useful tactic. Whole-grain snacks like oatmeal cookies, brown rice cakes, and whole-wheat crackers can be great selections. Because these complex carbohydrates take longer to break down, blood glucose is released gradually. Stable blood sugar levels are promoted by this constant energy source, which lessens the likelihood of spikes and crashes.

Including snacks high in protein is also crucial for maintaining energy levels and promoting muscular health. Snacks that are high in protein can include lean meats like chicken or turkey, Greek yogurt, or hard-boiled eggs. Protein is essential for satiety because it makes people feel fuller for longer periods and lessens their propensity to engage in unhealthy between-meal snacking.

Healthy fats also support long-term energy and general well-being. Foods like avocados, almonds, and seeds that are high in monounsaturated and polyunsaturated fats are good snack options. In addition to being a concentrated source of energy, these fats aid in the absorption of fat-soluble vitamins, so encouraging the best possible dietary intake.

Another crucial element of successful snacking tactics is hydration. Incorporating hydrated snacks, like slices of cucumber or watermelon, can improve general health and avoid dehydration, which is especially important for those who have an ileostomy.

People who have ileostomies should improve their snacking habits for sustained energy by combining complex carbohydrates, protein, healthy fats, and water. These techniques enhance mental and physical well-being in addition to supporting physical health.

Steer clear of problematic snack options:

When it comes to post-surgery nutrition for ostomates, staying away from unhealthy snack options is essential to preserving abdominal health and averting future issues. Even though it's important to have a range of snacks, some options may be difficult for people who have an ileostomy, so it's important to think things through carefully before choosing what to eat.

The avoidance of high-fiber snacks is one of the main things to think about. While too much fiber might be harmful to those who have an ileostomy, it is generally necessary for intestinal health. High-fiber snacks can be difficult to digest and cause discomfort or intestinal obstructions. Examples of these snacks are raw vegetables, entire nuts, and seeds. To reduce the chance of difficulties, people should choose cooked or peeled vegetables, nut butter, and seedless fruits.

Snacks with a lot of added sugar and artificial ingredients are another area to exercise caution. Excessive sugar intake may be a factor in digestive problems and inflammation.

A better option is to select snacks that have natural sugars, like those in fresh fruit. Furthermore, it's best to stay away from snacks that contain artificial coloring, preservatives, or sweeteners because they can irritate the digestive system and cause discomfort.

Additionally, processed and high-sodium snacks need to be handled carefully. These foods increase the risk of dehydration, which is especially dangerous for people who have an ileostomy.

A healthy balance can be maintained by choosing whole, minimally processed meals and by reading labels to check the sodium amount.

Carbonated drinks and some foods that cause gas should also be avoided because they might cause bloating and discomfort. Abdominal distension can be caused by gas-producing foods like beans and cruciferous vegetables as well as carbonated drinks that force extra air into the digestive tract.

In conclusion, it is critical for people with ileostomies to make educated decisions and to be aware of potentially problematic snack selections.

People can support abdominal wellness and reduce the risk of issues by avoiding high-fiber, sugary, processed, and gas-producing snacks. This will ensure a balanced and nourishing diet that is customized to meet each individual's needs.

CHAPTER TEN

SOCIALIZING AND EATING OUT

Tips for Dining at Restaurants

While eating out can be a fun event, people who have an ileostomy must take care to ensure that they enjoy themselves as well as follow their post-surgery dietary requirements. Finding a balance between enjoying delectable foods and preserving intestinal health is crucial.

Pre-researching the restaurant is an important piece of advice. Menus are frequently accessible online thanks to the internet, enabling people to determine whether the alternatives are appropriate. Selecting restaurants that offer a range of protein sources, cooked veggies, and easily digested grains is advantageous. Another crucial step is telling the server about your dietary restrictions. To meet your demands, they can help you navigate the menu, make suggestions for changes, or even communicate with the chef. Good communication keeps things running smoothly and avoids unforeseen problems during the eating experience.

Lean protein options on the menu, like grilled chicken or fish, are typically well-tolerated. Vegetables that have been steamed or sautéed and quickly digested starches like quinoa or rice make great sides. It is best to stay away from dishes that are really hot or highly seasoned because they can aggravate the digestive tract. Moderation is also essential; choose smaller servings and chew your meal well to facilitate digestion.

It's crucial to stay hydrated throughout meals because dehydration is a significant worry for those who have an ileostomy. However, since they may cause discomfort or gas, it's advisable to minimize or stay away from carbonated drinks and excessively sweetened liquids.

It's also very important to be organized. Having extra pouches and wipes for your ostomy means that any unforeseen problems can be handled discreetly. It's also crucial to have an optimistic outlook; don't let dietary limitations take away from the fun of sharing a meal with others. These suggestions can make eating out with an ileostomy pleasurable and stress-free, enhancing both mental and physical health.

Sharing Dietary Requirements

Navigating food demands after ileostomy surgery requires clear and effective communication, particularly when dining out or at social gatherings. It's critical to speak up for oneself and make sure people realize how important it is to follow certain dietary guidelines.

It is important to explain to friends, family, and restaurant staff the importance of the ileostomy diet for abdominal health. Giving a quick rundown of the procedure and how it affects digestion aids in others' understanding of why specific food selections are required. Stressing how following these recommendations immediately improves general comfort and health encourages compassion and understanding.

It's important to be upfront and truthful about dietary requirements in social settings. When friends and family are aware of certain constraints, they are frequently more than happy to make thoughtful accommodations. When you're invited to someone's party, for example, think about talking about possible menu items or even volunteering to bring food that fits the ileostomy diet. This proactive strategy promotes diversity throughout the social circle in addition to guaranteeing a safe and enjoyable dining experience.

It's important to tell the waitress about any dietary restrictions in a restaurant setting with confidence. All it takes is a subdued but explicit explanation of why a low-fiber, quickly-digested meal is necessary. Numerous dining establishments are experienced in accommodating different dietary requirements and can offer appropriate substitutes or adjustments. Having a courteous but firm stance on these demands promotes a cooperative and upbeat environment.

Effective communication is ultimately a two-way street. Although it's important to express one's needs clearly, a cooperative approach is shown by being open to suggestions or changes made by others. People who have an ileostomy can benefit from social connections without sacrificing their abdominal health if they are encouraged to communicate freely.

Managing Social Gatherings with A Certainty

After ileostomy surgery, navigating social situations with assurance requires a trifecta of readiness, assurance, and skillful communication. With the appropriate attitude and preparation, people with an ileostomy can completely participate in social activities, whether they are attending a wedding, a family reunion, or a casual get-together.

The first step in preparation is to have a complete grasp of the event. Making proactive decisions is made possible by being aware of the kind of food that will be provided. To make sure that appropriate options are available, it is best to get in touch with the host or organizer to discuss dietary requirements. A kind act that ensures a secure and satisfying dinner is offering to bring food that fits the ileostomy diet to the gathering.

Making the appropriate clothing selections is another factor. Choosing loose-fitting apparel can improve comfort and aid in discretely hiding the ostomy pouch. It's a good idea to fill a compact bag with necessary items like extra pouches, wipes, and odor-neutralizing products to be ready for any last-minute problems.

Gaining confidence requires constant work. Regaining confidence greatly depends on accepting one's body and the changes it has experienced. A sense of understanding and solidarity can be fostered by joining support groups or discussing experiences with close friends. Self-esteem can also be increased by emphasizing the benefits of social connections and the delight of being in the present.

The ability to communicate effectively is essential for navigating social situations. Ensuring that hosts or restaurant workers are aware of your dietary requirements guarantees that the right arrangements may be made. It can be useful to have a code or discrete signal with close friends or family to let them know when managing ostomy care requires a break or a private moment.

In conclusion, having preparedness, confidence, and skillful communication are all necessary for navigating social situations after ileostomy surgery. People may participate fully in social activities and promote a sense of normalcy and well-being by taking a proactive and upbeat stance.

CHAPTER ELEVEN

STOMA CARE AND MAINTENANCE

Proper Cleaning and Care Techniques for Ileostomy:

It is critical for the general comfort and well-being of those who have had ostomy surgery to maintain appropriate cleanliness and care for an ileostomy. Using the right cleaning methods to keep the area around the stoma clean and healthy is one of the most important parts of caring for a stoma.

It is essential to gather all required materials before beginning the cleaning process, including gauze or cotton balls, lukewarm water, and mild soap. To avoid cross-contamination throughout the cleaning process, start by giving yourself a thorough hand wash. Remove the ostomy pouch gently, being cautious not to overstretch the adhesive. Throw away the used pouch properly.

After that, wash the area surrounding the stoma with lukewarm water and gentle soap; stay away from abrasive chemicals or scented soaps that could irritate the skin. Using a gentle towel, pat the area dry or allow it to air dry naturally. It is imperative to refrain from using tissues or clothing that may stick to the stoma due to loose fibers.

While cleaning, keep an eye out for any odd changes in size or form, redness, or irritation around the stoma. A wet cotton ball or piece of gauze can be used to gently remove any crusts or dried discharge. Being gentle is crucial to avoid damaging the sensitive stoma tissue.

Apply a barrier to protect the skin from irritation after washing, such as stoma powder or paste, to assist keep the skin's seal intact when putting on a fresh ostomy pouch. Make sure the pouching system is properly fitted to avoid leaks and discomfort. An essential part of good cleaning and maintenance practices is replacing the pouch regularly and keeping an eye on the stoma's condition.

Being consistent is essential to keeping up with stoma care. Developing a regimen and following it religiously will help improve overall abdominal well-being and maintain a healthier stoma.

Identifying Concerning Signs in Ileostomy Patients:

For ileostomy patients to ensure optimal abdominal health and swiftly treat any potential concerns, they must remain vigilant about the signals of concern. People can identify issues early and take prompt action by being vigilant and aware of their stoma and the surroundings.

Keeping an eye out for changes in the stoma's appearance is essential to identifying warning indications. Any appreciable changes in size, color, or form could be a symptom of serious problems such as inflammation, infection, or a compromised blood supply. Any unexpected discharge, severe bleeding, or discoloration should be seen by medical specialists right once.

Ileostomy patients should be aware of any changes in their general well-being in addition to ocular assessment. Unusual feelings, persistent pain, or discomfort near the stoma site could indicate underlying issues. Bowel habit changes, including an abrupt rise in output or the onset of diarrhea, may also be signs of problems that need to be addressed.

Ostomates have to keep a close eye out for any indications of irritation, redness, or rashes on the skin around the stoma. Skin issues may be a sign of additional issues, such as allergies to ostomy supplies, or a poorly fitted pouch. When these problems are detected early on, stoma care practices and product choices can be modified.

Another area of concern for ileostomy care is odor management. Bad smells could be a sign of infection or leakage, which would call for a careful evaluation of the pouching system and stoma cleaning procedures. To avoid issues and promote abdominal wellness in ileostomy patients, they must maintain open communication with healthcare providers and seek early help when any indicators of worry occur.

Seeking Expert Guidance for Patients with Ileostomies:

Even though ileostomy patients are capable of handling many parts of their care on their own, consulting a physician is essential to preserving good abdominal well-being. For ileostomy patients, seeking advice from medical specialists—such as gastroenterologists and ostomy nurses—provides important assurance, direction, and individualized treatment strategies.

Frequent follow-up visits with medical professionals enable a thorough evaluation of the stoma's general health and well-being and the modification of care regimens as necessary. Ostomy nurses are essential in teaching stoma care skills, diagnosing and solving frequent problems, and suggesting appropriate items to improve comfort and effectiveness.

Ileostomy patients should not hesitate to seek expert help when experiencing new symptoms, worries, or difficulties relating to their stoma, in addition to routine check-ups. Whether the issue is with pouching systems, sudden odors, or changes in stool consistency, consulting healthcare professionals as soon as possible can guarantee rapid intervention and resolution.

Expert guidance is especially important for people getting used to living with an ileostomy. Healthcare professionals can help with body image issues, offer emotional support, and refer patients to support groups or counseling programs. Building a cooperative connection with medical staff gives ileostomy patients a sense of security and confidence, enabling them to successfully manage the difficulties of life after surgery.

To sum up, seeing a professional is not a show of weakness but rather a proactive move toward preserving the best possible abdominal well-being. The knowledge and direction that medical professionals offer greatly enhance the general health and well-being of those who have an ileostomy.

CHAPTER TWELVE

MENTAL AND EMOTIONAL WELLBEING

Coping with Body Image Changes

One's body image is significantly altered after ileostomy surgery, and managing these changes is essential for maintaining mental and emotional well. People could feel a variety of things, such as sadness, humiliation, or self-consciousness. Recognizing these feelings and realizing that they are perfectly normal responses to the changes in one's physical appearance is crucial. One of the most important aspects of coping is adopting a positive perspective regarding the altered body image.

Fostering self-acceptance and self-love is a necessary step in embracing a new self-image. Exercise and hobbies, which are activities that boost self-esteem, might assist in turning attention away from bodily changes and toward one's abilities and capabilities.

Joining ostomate support groups or seeking assistance from mental health specialists can offer a forum for exchanging experiences and picking up useful coping mechanisms. Concerns concerning one's body image should be discussed openly with healthcare professionals to receive helpful, individually tailored advice and guidance.

Looking into comfortable yet fashionable clothing options for ostomates can have a big impact on body image in addition to providing psychological support. The fashion industry has expanded its inclusivity by providing discreetly accommodating ostomy pouch-compatible clothes. Regaining confidence in one's appearance after surgery and cultivating a healthier mindset are two benefits of taking a proactive and positive approach to these changes.

Establishing a Network of Support

Having a strong support network is essential for overcoming the difficulties associated with having an ileostomy and has a positive impact on mental and emotional health.

The road following surgery can be emotionally exhausting, therefore it can be quite beneficial to have a support system of sympathetic and understanding people. Family members, close friends, other ostomates, or mental health specialists who specialize in helping people deal with significant life upheavals could make up this support network.

For a robust support system to be established, communication is essential. Understanding and empathy are fostered when ideas, worries, and victories are shared with those close to us. In addition to offering emotional support, loved ones can help people adjust to their new lifestyle by offering useful assistance. By eradicating myths and raising awareness, teaching close friends and family members about the mental and physical challenges of having an ileostomy helps create a more accepting atmosphere.

Participating in ostomate support groups provides a special forum for people to meet others going through comparable struggles. These support groups give a forum for exchanging coping mechanisms, experiences, and emotional support.

Local support organizations, community gatherings, and online forums are excellent places to meet new people and form deep relationships with people who are aware of the subtleties of living with an ileostomy.

Stress Reduction with Mindfulness

After ileostomy surgery, maintaining mental and emotional well-being for individuals requires a commitment to mindfulness and stress management practices. Stress can arise from adjusting to a new lifestyle and the possible difficulties that come with having an ileostomy. Deep breathing exercises and other mindfulness-based activities can help control stress and foster serenity.

People can cultivate a good mindset by integrating mindfulness into their everyday activities, which enables them to remain focused and present. By promoting acceptance of the present, mindfulness practices support overcoming obstacles with composure and clarity of thought. Stress-reduction and mindfulness-focused apps and guided sessions are widely accessible, providing people with easily integrated tools into their daily lives.

Stress treatment includes both lifestyle modifications and mindfulness. Keeping a balanced diet, getting regular exercise, and emphasizing self-care are all important for general well-being. Since sleep is essential for both physical and mental healing, getting enough of it is essential for stress management. To ensure that techniques are tailored to individual needs and health considerations, consulting with healthcare specialists is a good idea for individualized stress management approaches.

In conclusion, developing stress management strategies and embracing mindfulness practices are effective coping mechanisms for those managing their ileostomy. By fostering mental and emotional resilience, these techniques enable people to meet obstacles head-on with a good attitude and a sense of inner serenity.

CHAPTER THIRTEEN

TRAVELING WITH AN ILEOSTOMY

Planning for Travel Success:

Careful planning is essential when traveling with an ileostomy to guarantee a seamless and enjoyable stay. Understanding your unique nutritional requirements and preferences is the first step. Because of the nature of an ileostomy, patients need to be aware of their nutritional needs and steer clear of specific foods that could cause problems or discomfort. An essential step in the planning process is speaking with a healthcare provider to customize a diet plan for each person based on their unique medical needs.

Choosing suitable travel locations and lodging is crucial, in addition to nutritional considerations. Selecting locations with access to ostomy supplies and reputable medical facilities is advised. Important aspects of organizing a trip include learning about the availability of ostomy-friendly restrooms, researching local medical services, and being conscious of the climate and how it can affect your health.

Making sure you pack well is essential to a successful trip. Enough supplies, such as adhesive removers, ostomy bags, and hygiene items, ought to be packaged in large enough numbers. It is best to have extra supplies on hand in case there are unforeseen difficulties or delays. Keeping these materials organized in a special travel pouch makes them easier to reach and reduces the stress that comes with ileostomy management on the go.

Creating a travel schedule that allows for frequent rest periods and breaks is also essential. This lowers the chance of stress-related problems and helps manage energy levels in addition to enabling essential ostomy care. When required, let authorities or other travelers know about your medical condition to create a supportive environment for the duration of the trip.

In the end, careful planning is essential to an enjoyable and successful journey for those who have an ileostomy. When dietary requirements are taken care of, appropriate places are chosen, necessary supplies are packed, and a well-organized schedule is planned, travelers can travel with confidence, knowing that their health and well-being are top priorities.

Handling Supplies While Traveling:

The careful management of supplies is an essential part of traveling for those who have an ileostomy. A planned strategy for handling and packing ostomy supplies when traveling is essential to a smooth and successful trip.

First and foremost, you must determine how much supply you will need for the entire trip. This includes having a sufficient supply of adhesive products, cleaning wipes, ostomy bags, and any other particular supplies that medical specialists may advise. As a general guideline, you should bring at least 1.5 times your daily allowance to allow for unforeseen circumstances or lengthy trips.

Using a sturdy and safe travel pouch or organizer is advised to maintain the integrity of supplies. Things are kept in order in this specific area, which also shields them from harm and the elements. When packing, take the destination's climate into account. Extreme heat or humidity can affect the ostomy items' adhesive qualities.

It is important to review all travel limitations and laws, particularly when traveling between borders. Certain medical supplies may be restricted in some nations, or they may call for particular paperwork. Being knowledgeable about these factors guarantees a hassle-free travel experience and helps prevent issues at security checkpoints.

Having a backup plan for restocking goods while traveling is also safe. In the event of an emergency or unanticipated delay, knowing which pharmacies or medical supply businesses are nearby can be quite helpful. Furthermore, having a compact emergency kit in a carry-on bag with the necessary supplies allows for quick access when traveling.

To avoid leaks or discomfort, supplies must be regularly inspected and maintained during the trip. Organizing rest periods that enable covert ostomy care, especially on lengthy flights or road journeys, makes traveling more bearable.

All things considered, careful handling of ostomy equipment is essential to a smooth and worry-free trip. People with ileostomies can travel with confidence and put their health and well-being first by measuring quantities, employing secure storage, following travel laws, and making backup plans.

Handling Stress Associated with Travel:

Traveling may be stressful whether it is for work or pleasure, and for those who have an ileostomy, there may be more factors to worry about. However, stress may be reduced and the trip can be made as enjoyable as possible with careful planning and a proactive attitude.

The worry of not being well-prepared is one of the main things that stress out ostomates when they travel. Comprehensive planning is essential to combat this. This entails planning the appropriate medical supplies in addition to learning about the medical condition and informing fellow travelers about it. By fostering a supportive environment and sharing information with those around you, you can lessen the psychological stress of managing an ileostomy in unfamiliar environments.

Keeping your schedule flexible is another good way to reduce stress. Traveling may involve unforeseen events like airline delays or itinerary changes. An organized timetable that includes sabbaticals for relaxation and ostomy care acts as a safety net against unforeseen circumstances and reduces stress.

It is vital to integrate stress-reduction strategies into the travel regimen. Relaxation techniques like deep breathing, mindfulness, or meditation can ease anxiety and enhance well-being. When dealing with stressful situations like negotiating congested airports or unexpected delays, these approaches can be especially helpful.

Maintaining hydration and making nutrition a top priority is essential for general health, particularly when traveling. Stress levels might rise and physical health can be impacted by dehydration and unhealthful eating habits. Keeping a reusable water bottle with you and choosing healthy foods will help you stay energized and resilient to stress.

Enjoyable activities can also act as a diversion from certain tensions when traveling. Having entertainment alternatives close at hand might be a good way to decompress, whether it's through reading, listening to music, or viewing a favorite movie.

Finally, it's critical to recognize and respect any emotional responses to the difficulties of traveling while wearing an ileostomy. Asking friends, family, or online groups for support can provide insightful information and emotional support. It creates a sense of camaraderie and lessens feelings of loneliness to share experiences with people who comprehend the special difficulties involved with ostomy treatment.

Therefore, cautious planning, flexibility, stress-relieving methods, and emotional support are all necessary for managing travel-related stress when living with an ileostomy. By implementing these techniques, people can travel with confidence, concentrate on the good parts of the experience, and keep their well-being throughout the voyage.

CHAPTER FOURTEEN

LONG-TERM OSTOMY CARE

Regular Check-ups and Monitoring

After ileostomy surgery, long-term ostomy care entails a careful schedule of routine examinations and monitoring to guarantee the ongoing health of those who have an ostomy. Following surgery, medical professionals are essential in assisting ostomates in overcoming the difficulties of this new way of life. Regular check-ups are crucial to determining the state of the stoma, assessing the person's general health, and handling any potential issues or consequences.

Healthcare specialists meticulously inspect the stoma at these scheduled checkups, searching for indications of discomfort, infection, or any changes in size or color. They also check the surrounding skin for any indications of dermatological problems to preserve the abdominal well-being of the ostomate. Another important factor is to keep an eye on the stoma's output, as this can reveal information about how well the digestive system is working and signal possible problems like dehydration or food allergies.

Regular check-ups provide ostomates with opportunities to talk about their emotional and psychological well-being in addition to the physical checkup. Living with an ostomy can be a life-changing experience, but long-term adaption requires resolving the difficulties and adaptations that come with it. To promote a comprehensive approach to ostomy care, healthcare professionals can provide advice on managing anxiety, body image problems, and other social concerns.

For those with an ostomy, self-monitoring is advised in addition to consulting with a healthcare specialist. Ostomates who have mastered the art of body signal observation and interpretation are more equipped to participate actively in their long-term care. People who maintain a stoma diary can record dietary changes, regularity of output, and any possible problems. This information can be very helpful when visiting a doctor. Thus, self-monitoring and routine check-ups foster a cooperative relationship between ostomates and medical professionals, enabling thorough and individualized care that caters to each patient's particular needs.

Adjusting Over Time to Changes

A key component of long-term ostomy care is helping patients adjust to changing circumstances as their post-surgery lifestyles change over time. In addition to physical adjustments, ostomates must also make mental and social adjustments. For this reason, they must learn to be resilient and adaptable in their outlook on life.

Over time, the stoma's physical dimensions may change, requiring modifications to the kind and dimensions of ostomy appliances. The risk of leaks and skin irritation is reduced with a suitable fit guaranteed by routine reevaluation of the ostomy equipment. The characteristics of the stoma can be affected by changes in body weight, activities, or age-related factors, highlighting the necessity for continual adaptation.

Overcoming early obstacles and accepting a new sense of normalcy are essential steps in adjusting emotionally and socially to live with an ostomy. Ostomates frequently go through an adjustment phase during which they learn how to handle issues with their bodies, their self-worth, and their relationships. Education, counseling, and support groups are essential in helping people adjust to these changes and build a sense of understanding and community.

Furthermore, the ever-improving quality of life for ostomates is facilitated by the growing nature of medical technologies and ostomy care products. Keeping up with the most recent developments enables people to make knowledgeable decisions regarding their care, guaranteeing they take advantage of breakthroughs that improve convenience and comfort.

At the end of the day, being able to adjust to changes over time is a dynamic process that calls for constant learning, introspection, and a proactive attitude toward one's well-being. Long-term ostomy care is a journey that requires constant adaptation to the life circumstances of an ostomate, which is not a static idea.

Honoring Recovery Milestones

Numerous benchmarks are encountered during long-term ostomy care; each one signifies a victory over difficulties and a stride toward long-term well-being. Honoring these anniversaries is not only a symbolic gesture; it is also an essential part of cultivating optimism and bolstering the fortitude of those who have had ileostomy surgery.

The accomplishment of successfully adjusting to daily life with an ostomy is one noteworthy milestone. Following surgery, there is frequently a learning curve over the first few weeks as people get used to controlling the stoma, switching appliances, and taking care of any potential issues. Celebrating your success in mastering these useful skills helps you feel accomplished and more confident.

The capacity to keep up a healthy, balanced diet is another important turning point. After ileostomy surgery, patients may experience difficulties and limitations with food at first. Regaining control over these challenges and progressively adding more diversity to the diet is an impressive accomplishment. Long-term ostomy care depends heavily on nutrition, which affects general health and well-being. Honoring the capacity to partake in a varied and balanced diet demonstrates the person's dedication to self-care and underscores the beneficial influence on their life quality.

Another significant turning point in the healing process is social reintegration. Taking part in relationships, hobbies, and community service helps to break down any barriers that one may have placed on oneself and promotes a sense of normalcy. Honoring the capacity to engage fully in social life serves to reaffirm that having an ostomy does not have to be a barrier to development; rather, it may be a source of strength, resiliency, and a fresh sense of purpose in life.

In addition, achieving psychological benchmarks is essential to long-term ostomy treatment. Resolving emotions of guilt, stigma, or seclusion is a significant accomplishment. A community that is encouraging and empowering is enriched by celebrating the growth of a positive self-image, sound mental health, and the capacity to share experiences with others.

Fundamentally, commemorating recovery milestones is an acknowledgment of the ostomate's fortitude, tenacity, and capacity to face life with fortitude. These occasions act as inspirational catalysts for the continuous process of long-term ostomy care, in addition to being indicators of accomplishment.

CHAPTER FIFTEEN

CONCLUSION AND EMPOWERMENT

Reflecting on Your Journey:

Before beginning, it's crucial to take a moment to consider your post-ileostomy surgery nutrition path. Consider the perseverance and fortitude you've displayed throughout the project. You have undoubtedly bravely and devotedly surmounted numerous obstacles, from the challenges of surgery to acclimating to a new way of life. Reflecting on your journey will help you appreciate and acknowledge the improvements you've made, both mentally and physically.

Jot down the dietary adjustments you've made and the advantages they've given your digestive system. Enjoy the moments when you can balance your food to provide your body with the nutrition it requires with the least bit of discomfort. Looking back on your path might also help you identify areas where you could still be adjusting or learning.

This offers an opportunity for understanding and self-empathy, recognizing that regaining optimal nutrition following ileostomy is a lifelong, constantly evolving process.

As you reflect, consider keeping a journal to document your experiences, setbacks, and victories. This can be a helpful tool for self-improvement and may provide some perspective for individuals in the ostomy community who are going through similar things. You make room for continued growth and empowerment by being self-aware and reflecting.

Choosing a Joyful and Healthful Way of Life:

Adopting a happy and healthy lifestyle after ileostomy surgery entails more than just dietary choices; it entails a comprehensive approach to well-being. As you navigate this new chapter of your life, remember to prioritize your emotional, social, and physical well-being. Engage in pleasurable pursuits that improve your overall health.

Physical well-being depends on doing frequent exercise that fits your talents and comfort level. Consult with medical professionals to choose suitable activities that improve overall health and abdominal strength. It's normal to be concerned about keeping a healthy weight. You can achieve and sustain this goal with the support of a well-balanced diet and consistent exercise.

Emotional well-being holds equal significance. Create a support system of friends, family, or other ostomates who can relate to and understand your situation. Seek professional therapy if necessary, as coping with the emotional challenges of living with an ileostomy may require special support.

Furthermore, nourish your mind with knowledge. Stay up to date on the latest advancements in ostomy care, abdominal wellness, and dietary recommendations. Through education, you become more empowered and are more equipped to advocate for yourself within the healthcare system.

Encouraging People in the Ostomy Community:

Your knowledge of post-ileostomy nutrition and abdominal health makes you a role model for the ostomy community. When sharing your successes, failures, and experiences, be truthful and open. Those going through a similar scenario could get inspiration and a sense of support from your story.

Connecting with other ostomates through online forums or support groups can facilitate the exchange of words of wisdom and encouragement. We are all empowered by sharing our stories with others in a way that transcends our individual experiences. Not only should one highlight accomplishments but also acknowledge failures and offer guidance on overcoming them to motivate others.

To get more readers and spread the word about your message, start a blog or use social media platforms. Beyond personal connections, the greater ostomy community can benefit from your activism. In addition to bolstering others' resilience and sense of purpose, encouraging others builds a mutually beneficial relationship that unifies and strengthens the ostomy community.

Post-ileostomy empowerment, to put it briefly, entails a range of interconnected actions, including reflecting on your experience, embracing a healthy lifestyle, and inspiring others in the ostomy community.

As you travel this path, remember that your stories not only demonstrate your tenacity but also provide encouragement and support to those who may be embarking on their journey toward abdominal wellness after surgery.

BONUS SECTION

23 Quick and Simple Illustrated Healing Recipes + Preparatory Procedures For Ostomates Nutritional Wellness

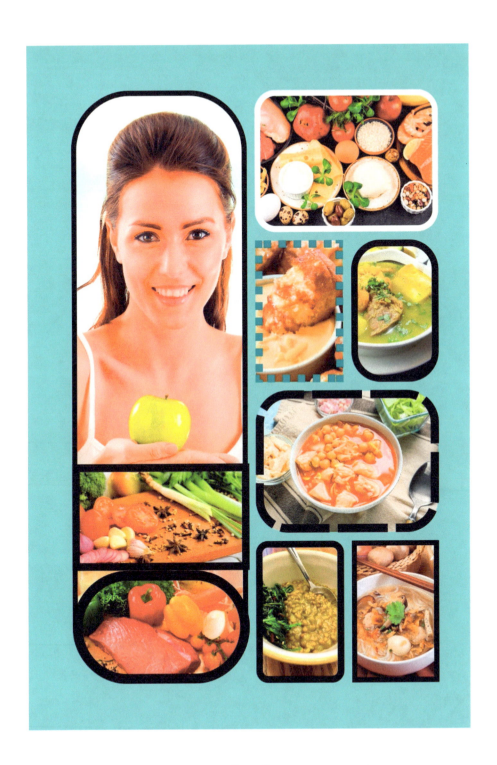

RECIPE 1:

SOOTHING SMOOTHIE BOWL

Preparatory and Instruction Guidelines for Soothing Smoothie Bowl (Ileostomy Diet)

Introduction:

Following ileostomy surgery, it is crucial to adopt a nutrient-rich diet that supports abdominal wellness. The Soothing Smoothie Bowl is an excellent addition to the ileostomy diet, providing a blend of soothing ingredients that are gentle on the digestive system. This quick and simple recipe features bananas, Greek yogurt, honey, and almond milk, offering a creamy and nutritious option for ostomates.

Preparation Guidelines:

1. **Gather Ingredients:**

• Ensure you have ripe bananas, high-quality Greek yogurt (preferably low-fat), pure honey, and unsweetened almond milk.

- Choose soft fruits for topping, such as berries or sliced kiwi, to add extra nutrition and texture.

2. Kitchen Hygiene:

- Wash your hands thoroughly before handling any ingredients to maintain a sterile environment, especially crucial for individuals recovering from surgery.

3. Equipment Preparation:

- Check that your blender is clean and sanitized. Run it through a quick rinse if needed.

- Have a spatula, measuring cups, and a bowl ready for assembling and serving.

Instructions:

1. Peeling and Slicing:

- Peel and slice the ripe bananas into smaller chunks. This ensures smoother blending.

2. Measuring Ingredients:

- Measure the desired amount of Greek yogurt, honey, and almond milk. Adjust quantities based on personal taste preferences and nutritional requirements.

3. Blending Process:

•   Place the banana slices, Greek yogurt, honey, and a splash of almond milk into the blender.

•   Blend the ingredients on a low setting initially to avoid splashing. Gradually increase the speed until you achieve a smooth and creamy consistency.

4. Texture Adjustment:

•   Assess the texture of the smoothie. If it's too thick, add a bit more almond milk and blend again until the desired consistency is reached.

5. Taste Test:

•   Taste the smoothie mixture and adjust sweetness by adding more honey if necessary. Ensure it meets your flavor preferences.

6. Serving:

•   Pour the smoothie into a bowl, ensuring a smooth and even surface.

7. Topping Arrangement:

•   Garnish the smoothie bowl with soft fruits like berries or sliced kiwi. These not only add a burst of flavor but also provide additional vitamins and antioxidants.

8. Enjoy Mindfully:

•   Consume the Soothing Smoothie Bowl slowly and mindfully, savoring each spoonful. Chew thoroughly to aid digestion.

Additional Tips:

•   Temperature Consideration:

•   For those with sensitivity to cold foods, let the smoothie bowl sit at room temperature for a few minutes before consumption.

•   Hydration:

•   Accompany the smoothie bowl with small sips of water to stay adequately hydrated.

•   Customization:

- Experiment with other soft fruits or add a sprinkle of chia seeds for added texture and nutritional benefits.

By following these preparatory and instructional guidelines, individuals on an ileostomy diet can enjoy a delicious and nutritious Soothing Smoothie Bowl that supports their post-surgery nutritional needs while being gentle on the digestive system.

RECIPE 2:

HEALING CHICKEN BROTH

When preparing Healing Chicken Broth for an Ileostomy Diet, it's crucial to focus on ingredients that are gentle on the digestive system while promoting healing. Here are detailed preparatory and instructional guidelines for this nourishing broth:

Ingredients:

1.   **Boiled Chicken**: Choose boneless, skinless chicken breasts or thighs. These are lean sources of protein that are easier to digest. Ensure the chicken is well-cooked to avoid any risk of infection.

2.   **Carrots:** Peel and chop carrots into small, bite-sized pieces. Carrots provide vitamins and minerals and add a subtle sweetness to the broth. Make sure they are well-cooked to enhance digestibility.

3.   **Celery:** Trim and chop celery stalks into small pieces. Celery is rich in antioxidants and can add a

refreshing flavor to the broth. Chopping it finely will help in easier digestion.

4.   **Rice:** Opt for white rice as it is generally easier on the digestive system compared to brown rice. Rinse the rice thoroughly to remove excess starch, making it gentler on the stomach.

Preparation Instructions:

1.   **Prepare the Chicken:**

•   In a large pot, place the chicken pieces and cover them with water.

•   Bring the water to a boil and then reduce the heat to a simmer.

•   Cook the chicken thoroughly until it's no longer pink in the center. This usually takes around 20-30 minutes.

2.   **Add Vegetables:**

•   Once the chicken is cooked, add the chopped carrots and celery to the pot.

• Continue simmering until the vegetables are tender. This helps in preserving the nutrients and making them easily digestible.

3. Incorporate Rice:

• Add the rinsed white rice to the broth. The rice will absorb the flavors and provide a soft texture to the broth.

4. Simmering:

• Allow the broth to simmer on low heat for an additional 15-20 minutes. This ensures that all the ingredients are well-cooked and the flavors are infused.

5. Seasoning:

• Keep the seasoning simple. Add a pinch of salt for taste, but be mindful of sodium levels, especially if advised by a healthcare professional.

6. Cooling and Storing:

• Once the broth is ready, let it cool before consuming. This prevents any burns or discomfort.

- Store the broth in airtight containers in the refrigerator for easy reheating. Make sure to remove any excess fat that solidifies on the surface after refrigeration.

Additional Tips:

- Drink the broth warm but not too hot to avoid irritation.

- Portion the broth into smaller servings for easy consumption.

- Consider consulting with a healthcare professional or a nutritionist to tailor the recipe to individual dietary needs.

This Healing Chicken Broth provides essential nutrients and is gentle on the stomach, making it a nourishing choice for individuals on an Ileostomy Diet during the post-surgery phase.

RECIPE 3

GENTLE GREEN PUREE

Preparing a Gentle Green Puree for an ileostomy diet requires careful consideration of the ingredients and the cooking method. Here are detailed preparatory and instructional guidelines for creating this healing recipe:

Preparatory and Instruction Guidelines

Ingredients:

- Spinach

- Zucchini

- Potato

Tools and Equipment:

- Steamer or steam basket

- Blender or food processor

- Pot for boiling (if needed)

Preparation Steps:

1.   Select Fresh Ingredients:

•   Choose fresh, organic vegetables to ensure the purity of the ingredients.

•   Wash the spinach thoroughly, removing any dirt or debris.

•   Peel and wash the zucchini and potato.

2.   Prep Vegetables:

•   Cut the zucchini and potato into small, uniform chunks. This ensures even cooking and blending.

•   For the spinach, remove any tough stems to enhance the smooth texture of the puree.

3.   Steaming Process:

•   Place the zucchini and potato chunks in a steamer or steam basket.

•   Steam the vegetables until they are tender. This usually takes about 8-10 minutes, but the exact time may vary depending on the size of the chunks and the steaming method used.

•   Add the spinach to the steamer during the last 2-3 minutes of cooking. This prevents overcooking and helps retain the vibrant green color.

4.   Cooling:

•   Allow the steamed vegetables to cool for a few minutes before blending. This prevents steam from building up in the blender, reducing the risk of burns.

5.   Blending Process:

•   Transfer the steamed vegetables to a blender or food processor.

•   Blend until you achieve a smooth and creamy consistency. If the mixture is too thick, you can add a small amount of water or a mild broth to reach the desired texture.

6.   Check Texture:

•   Ensure the puree is smooth and free of any fibrous bits that could be difficult for the digestive system to handle.

7.   Storage:

•   If you're preparing the puree in advance, store it in airtight containers in the refrigerator. Use it within a few days for optimal freshness and nutritional value.

8.   Serving Suggestions:

•   Serve the Gentle Green Puree at room temperature to make it more palatable.

•   Consider adding a dash of olive oil or a dollop of plain yogurt for extra flavor and moisture.

9.   Monitor Digestive Response:

•   Introduce the puree gradually into your diet and monitor how your digestive system responds. If any discomfort or irritation occurs, consult with your healthcare provider.

10.   Adapt to Personal Preferences:

•   Feel free to adjust the ratios of ingredients based on personal preferences and dietary tolerances.

By following these detailed preparatory and instructional guidelines, you can create a nutrient-packed and easily digestible Gentle Green Puree, tailored to the needs of an ileostomy diet for post-surgery nutrition and abdominal wellness.

RECIPE 4

EASY-TO-DIGEST OATMEAL

Here are detailed preparatory and instructional guidelines for this healing recipe:

Preparatory Guidelines:

1.   **Selecting Ingredients:**

•   Rolled Oats: Opt for high-quality, unprocessed rolled oats. They are rich in soluble fiber, which aids digestion and helps regulate bowel movements.

•   Mashed Banana: Choose ripe bananas, as they are easier to digest and add natural sweetness to the oatmeal. Bananas also provide potassium, an essential electrolyte often lost after surgery.

•   Cinnamon: This spice not only adds a delicious flavor but also has anti-inflammatory properties, contributing to abdominal wellness.

2.   Consider Dietary Restrictions:

•   Confirm any dietary restrictions or preferences the individual may have. Ensure the ingredients align with their specific dietary needs post-ileostomy surgery.

3.   Portion Control:

•   Measure the ingredients carefully to avoid overloading the dish. Smaller, controlled portions are easier on the digestive system.

Instructional Guidelines:

1.   Cooking the Oats:

•   Measure Oats: Begin by measuring the desired amount of rolled oats based on individual preferences and dietary requirements.

•   Combine Ingredients: In a saucepan, combine the measured oats with water or a suitable liquid (e.g., lactose-free milk) for added creaminess.

•   Cooking Time: Cook the oats over low to medium heat, stirring frequently. Be cautious not to overcook, as a softer consistency is easier to digest.

• Adjust Liquid: Adjust the liquid content based on preference. Some individuals may prefer a thicker consistency, while others may prefer a thinner texture.

2. Adding Mashed Banana:

• Select Ripe Bananas: Mash ripe bananas separately until smooth. Ripe bananas are not only easier to mash but also gentler on the digestive system.

• Incorporate into Oats: Add the mashed banana into the cooking oats and stir well. This not only enhances flavor but also contributes to the overall nutritional content.

3. Sprinkle Cinnamon:

• Select High-Quality Cinnamon: Use ground cinnamon of good quality for optimal flavor and health benefits.

• Sprinkle to Taste: Add a sprinkle of cinnamon to the oatmeal, adjusting to taste. Cinnamon not only adds warmth but also has potential anti-inflammatory properties beneficial for abdominal wellness.

4. Monitoring Consistency:

•   Observation: Keep a close eye on the consistency of the oatmeal. It should be soft and easily chewable, ensuring ease of digestion.

5. Serve Warm:

•   Serve Promptly: Once the oatmeal reaches the desired consistency, promptly remove it from heat and serve while warm. Warm foods are generally gentler on the digestive system.

By following these preparatory and instructional guidelines, you can create a nourishing and easy-to-digest oatmeal dish suitable for individuals on an ileostomy diet.

RECIPE 5

AVOCADO AND COTTAGE CHEESE MASH

Preparing Avocado and Cottage Cheese Mash for an ileostomy diet involves minimal effort, and the result is a delicious, nutrient-packed snack that is easy on the digestive system. Here are detailed preparatory and instruction guidelines:

Ingredients:

• **Mashed Avocado:** Choose a ripe avocado, as it will be easier to mash. Peel and pit the avocado, then mash it in a bowl using a fork or spoon until smooth.

• **Cottage Cheese:** Opt for low-fat or fat-free cottage cheese for a lighter option. Measure the desired amount based on your dietary preferences and nutritional needs.

• Lemon: A hint of lemon adds a refreshing zing to the mash. Use fresh lemon juice for the best flavor.

Preparatory Guidelines:

1. Choose Fresh Ingredients:

• Ensure that the avocado is ripe but not overly soft. A ripe avocado should yield slightly to gentle pressure but still feel firm.

• Check the expiry date of the cottage cheese and choose a fresh, unexpired container.

• Use a fresh lemon for the juice.

2. Prepare the Avocado:

• Cut the avocado in half, remove the pit, and scoop out the flesh with a spoon.

• Place the avocado in a bowl for mashing.

3. Mashing the Avocado:

• Use a fork or spoon to mash the avocado until it reaches a smooth consistency.

- If you prefer a chunkier texture, mash the avocado to your desired level.

4.   Add Cottage Cheese:

- Measure the desired amount of cottage cheese and add it to the mashed avocado.

- Gently fold the cottage cheese into the mashed avocado until well combined.

5.   Incorporate Lemon:

- Squeeze a small amount of fresh lemon juice into the mixture. Start with a little and adjust according to your taste preferences.

- The lemon not only adds flavor but can also help prevent the avocado from browning.

6.   Mix Thoroughly:

- Stir the ingredients thoroughly to ensure an even distribution of flavors.

Instruction Guidelines:

1.   Serve Immediately or Refrigerate:

•   Avocado can oxidize and turn brown over time. For the freshest taste, consume the mash immediately after preparation.

•   If you need to store it, cover the bowl with plastic wrap, pressing it directly against the surface of the mash to minimize air exposure. Refrigerate for short periods, and consume within a day or two.

2.   Pairing Options:

•   Enjoy the Avocado and Cottage Cheese Mash on its own as a snack or spread it on whole grain crackers or toast.

•   Consider adding a sprinkle of herbs or a pinch of salt and pepper for extra flavor.

3.   Adjust Consistency:

- If the mash is too thick, you can add a small amount of water, milk, or additional lemon juice to achieve the desired consistency.

4. Listen to Your Body:

- Pay attention to how your body responds to the snack. If any discomfort or digestive issues arise, consider adjusting the proportions or excluding specific ingredients based on your tolerance.

This Avocado and Cottage Cheese Mash is not only easy to prepare but also a great source of healthy fats and protein, making it a nourishing option for individuals on an ileostomy diet.

RECIPE 6

SOFT SCRAMBLED EGGS WITH SPINACH

Soft Scrambled Eggs with Spinach is a quick and simple healing recipe that provides a protein-packed option that is easy to digest and rich in essential nutrients. Follow these preparatory and instruction guidelines to ensure a nourishing and gentle meal:

Preparatory Guidelines:

1.   Wash Hands Thoroughly:

•   Before handling any ingredients, ensure that you wash your hands thoroughly with soap and water to maintain hygiene and prevent contamination.

2.   Choose Fresh Ingredients:

• Select fresh, high-quality eggs and spinach. Fresh ingredients contribute to the overall nutritional value of the meal.

3. Prepare Cooking Utensils:

• Gather necessary utensils, such as a non-stick skillet, spatula, and a mixing bowl. A non-stick skillet is ideal for easy cooking and cleaning.

4. Ensure a Clean Cooking Environment:

• Wipe down the cooking area to create a clean and sanitized workspace, minimizing the risk of bacterial contamination.

Instruction Guidelines:

1. Crack Eggs into a Mixing Bowl:

• Crack the required number of eggs into a mixing bowl. Using fresh eggs enhances the flavor and nutritional content.

2. Whisk Eggs Gently:

•   Whisk the eggs gently with a fork or whisk. Avoid excessive whisking to maintain a softer texture in the final dish.

3.   Prepare Spinach:

•   Rinse the spinach thoroughly under cold water. Pat it dry with paper towels. Remove any tough stems to ensure a tender and easily digestible texture.

4.   Sauté Spinach:

•   Heat a non-stick skillet over low-medium heat. Add a tiny bit of butter or olive oil. Sauté the spinach until it wilts, stirring occasionally. This step adds valuable nutrients without compromising digestibility.

5.   Add Whisked Eggs:

•   Once the spinach is wilted, pour the whisked eggs into the skillet. Stir gently to incorporate the spinach into the eggs. Continue stirring to achieve soft scrambled eggs.

6.   Control Cooking Temperature:

• Keep the heat low to prevent overcooking and to maintain the softness of the eggs. This ensures easy digestion for individuals with an ileostomy.

7. Season Mildly:

• Season the scrambled eggs with a pinch of salt and pepper to enhance flavor. Avoid using excessive spices or seasonings that may be harsh on the digestive system.

8. Serve Warm:

• Once the eggs are cooked to a soft consistency, transfer them to a plate. Serve the Soft Scrambled Eggs with Spinach warm to make it more palatable and enjoyable.

9. Monitor Portion Sizes:

• Pay attention to portion sizes, as smaller, more frequent meals can be beneficial for individuals with an ileostomy. Adjust serving sizes according to your personal nutritional needs.

10. Stay Hydrated:

• Accompany the meal with plenty of fluids to stay hydrated, aiding digestion and overall well-being.

By following these preparatory and instruction guidelines, you can create a nourishing Soft Scrambled Eggs with Spinach dish that aligns with the dietary considerations of individuals post-ileostomy surgery. This meal provides essential nutrients while being gentle on the digestive system, promoting abdominal wellness and recovery.

RECIPE 7

MASHED SWEET POTATOES WITH GINGER

Preparing Mashed Sweet Potatoes with Ginger can be a delicious and nutritious addition to an ileostomy diet, providing a soft and easily digestible option for individuals recovering from abdominal surgery. Follow these preparatory guidelines to ensure a quick and simple healing recipe:

Preparatory Guidelines:

1. Choose Fresh and Quality Ingredients:

• Select sweet potatoes that are firm, free of bruises, and have a vibrant color.

• Opt for fresh ginger, ensuring it is firm and without any signs of mold.

2. Clean and Peel the Sweet Potatoes:

• Wash the sweet potatoes thoroughly under running water to remove any dirt or debris.

•   Peel the sweet potatoes using a vegetable peeler to eliminate any tough or fibrous skin.

3. Cut into Uniform Pieces:

•   Cut the peeled sweet potatoes into uniform-sized pieces. This helps in even cooking and ensures a consistent texture when mashed.

4. Boil the Sweet Potatoes:

•   Place the sweet potato pieces in a pot and cover them with water.

•   Add a pinch of salt to enhance flavor.

•   Boil the sweet potatoes until they are fork-tender. This typically takes around 15-20 minutes.

5. Drain and Cool:

•   Once the sweet potatoes are cooked, drain the water and let them cool for a few minutes. This makes them easier to handle and prevents burns during the mashing process.

6. Mash with a Touch of Ginger:

• Transfer the boiled sweet potatoes to a mixing bowl.

• Add a small amount of freshly grated or minced ginger. Start with a teaspoon and adjust according to taste preferences.

• Mash the sweet potatoes and ginger together using a potato masher or a fork until you achieve a smooth consistency.

7. Adjust Seasoning:

• Taste the mashed sweet potatoes and adjust the seasoning if necessary. You can add a pinch of salt or a dash of pepper according to your liking.

8. Serve Warm:

• Serve the Mashed Sweet Potatoes with Ginger while they are still warm to maximize flavor and comfort.

9. Consider Texture Modifications:

• For individuals with specific dietary needs, you can adjust the texture by adding a little liquid (broth, milk, or a dairy-free alternative) to achieve the desired consistency.

10. Store or Freeze for Later:

•   If preparing ahead, store the mashed sweet potatoes in an airtight container in the refrigerator. Reheat as needed.

•   You can also freeze portions for later use, making it convenient for individuals managing an ileostomy.

By following these preparatory guidelines, you can create a nourishing and easy-to-digest Mashed Sweet Potatoes with Ginger side dish that aligns with the nutritional needs of those on an ileostomy diet, promoting abdominal wellness and aiding in the post-surgery recovery process.

RECIPE 8

SIMPLE QUINOA PORRIDGE

Preparing Simple Quinoa Porridge for individuals following an ileostomy diet involves careful consideration of ingredients and cooking methods to ensure it is both nutritious and gentle on the digestive system. Below are detailed preparatory and instructional guidelines:

Preparatory Guidelines:

1. Selecting Ingredients:

• **Quinoa:** Opt for white quinoa as it is generally easier to digest. Rinse it thoroughly before cooking to remove the bitter coating called saponin.

- **Almond Milk:** Choose unsweetened and fortified almond milk. It provides a creamy texture without adding unnecessary sugars.

- **Honey:** Use raw, unprocessed honey sparingly for a touch of sweetness. Ensure it's free from additives.

2. Cooking Quinoa:

- **Rinsing:** Rinse one cup of quinoa under cold water to remove saponin.

- **Cooking Method:** Combine quinoa with two cups of almond milk in a saucepan. Bring it to a boil, then reduce heat, cover, and simmer until quinoa is tender (usually around 15 minutes).

- **Stirring:** Stir occasionally to prevent sticking and ensure even cooking.

- **Consistency:** Adjust the almond milk quantity to achieve the desired porridge consistency.

3. Adding Honey:

- **Timing:** Add honey once the quinoa is fully cooked, just before serving.

- **Quantity:** Start with a small amount and adjust according to taste preferences.

Instruction Guidelines:

1. Cooking Process:

- Begin by rinsing the quinoa thoroughly under cold water.

- In a saucepan, combine 1 cup of quinoa with 2 cups of almond milk.

- Bring the mixture to a boil over medium heat.

- Once boiling, reduce the heat to low, cover the saucepan, and let it simmer for approximately 15 minutes or until the quinoa is tender.

- Stir occasionally to prevent sticking and ensure even cooking.

2. Adjusting Consistency:

•	Monitor the consistency of the porridge during the cooking process.

•	If the porridge becomes too thick, add more almond milk gradually until the desired consistency is achieved.

•	Keep in mind that the porridge will thicken slightly as it cools.

3. Sweetening with Honey:

•	After the quinoa is fully cooked, add a touch of honey to the porridge.

•	Start with a small amount and adjust based on individual sweetness preferences.

•	Stir the honey into the porridge until well combined.

4. Serving and Enjoying:

- Once the porridge reaches the desired consistency and sweetness, remove it from the heat.

- Allow it to cool slightly before serving.

- Serve the quinoa porridge warm, and if desired, top it with additional almond milk or fresh fruit for added flavor and nutritional benefits.

Additional Tips:

- **Variations:** Explore variations by adding sliced bananas, berries, or a sprinkle of cinnamon for added flavor.

- **Texture Preferences:** Adjust the cooking time and almond milk quantity based on personal texture preferences.

- **Portion Control:** Be mindful of portion sizes to avoid overeating, especially for those with sensitive digestive systems.

This Simple Quinoa Porridge is not only easy to prepare but also provides a nourishing option for individuals on an ileostomy diet, promoting abdominal wellness and post-surgery nutrition.

RECIPE 9

BAKED SALMON WITH LEMON

This Baked Salmon with Lemon recipe is not only delicious but also rich in omega-3 fatty acids, providing essential nutrients for your post-surgery nutrition. Here are detailed preparatory and instruction guidelines to ensure a safe and nourishing meal for individuals with an ileostomy:

Preparatory Guidelines:
1.   **Select Fresh Salmon:**

- Choose fresh, high-quality salmon fillets. Fresh fish is essential for both flavor and nutritional content.

- Ensure the salmon has been properly cleaned and deboned to avoid any discomfort during digestion.

2. Consider Ileostomy-Friendly Seasonings:

- Opt for seasonings that are gentle on the digestive system. Lemon, herbs like dill or parsley, and mild spices can enhance the flavor without irritating.

3. Preheat Oven:

- Preheat your oven to a moderate temperature, typically around 375°F (190°C). This ensures even cooking and a perfectly baked salmon.

4. Prepare a Non-Stick Baking Dish:

- Use a non-stick baking dish or line a regular dish with parchment paper to prevent the salmon from sticking. This makes it easier to handle and reduces the risk of added fats or oils.

Instruction Guidelines:

1. Season the Salmon:

• Gently pat the salmon fillets dry with paper towels. Season both sides with a pinch of salt and pepper.

• Optionally, add a squeeze of fresh lemon juice over the fillets. Lemon not only enhances the flavor but also aids digestion.

2.   Place Salmon in Baking Dish:

• Arrange the seasoned salmon fillets in the prepared baking dish, leaving enough space between each piece for even cooking.

3.   Bake in Preheated Oven:

• Place the baking dish in the preheated oven and bake for approximately 15-20 minutes, or until the salmon is cooked through and flakes easily with a fork.

4.   Monitor Cooking Time:

• Keep a close eye on the salmon to avoid overcooking. Cooking times may vary depending on the thickness of the fillets, so adjust accordingly.

5.   Serve with a Side of Lemon:

•   Once baked, remove the salmon from the oven and let it rest for a few minutes. Serve with an additional squeeze of fresh lemon juice for added brightness.

6.   Think About Complements:

•   Pair the baked salmon with ileostomy-friendly sides such as steamed vegetables, white rice, or mashed potatoes for a well-balanced and easily digestible meal.

Additional Tips:

•   Portion Control:

•   Pay attention to portion sizes to prevent overeating and to ensure that the meal is well-tolerated by your digestive system.

•   Stay Hydrated:

•   Drink an adequate amount of water throughout the meal and after to maintain hydration and support digestion.

By following these preparatory and instruction guidelines, you can enjoy a delicious and nutritionally beneficial Baked Salmon with Lemon while prioritizing your abdominal wellness in an ileostomy diet. Always consult with your healthcare provider or a registered dietitian for personalized dietary recommendations based on your specific health needs.

RECIPE 10

CUCUMBER AND MINT INFUSED WATER

Here's a detailed set of preparatory or instruction guidelines for making Cucumber and Mint Infused Water, keeping in mind the needs of an ileostomy diet and post-surgery nutrition for abdominal wellness:

Preparation Guidelines for Cucumber and Mint-Infused Water:

1. Select Fresh and High-Quality Ingredients:

•   Choose fresh and firm cucumbers for slicing. Organic cucumbers are preferable, especially if the skin is included.

•   Pick fresh mint leaves with a vibrant green color and a strong aroma.

2. Wash and Sanitize:

•   Thoroughly wash the cucumbers and mint leaves under cold running water to remove any dirt or contaminants.

•   Sanitize your cutting board, knife, and any other utensils used in the preparation to maintain a sterile environment.

3. Peel and Slice the Cucumbers:

•   If your ileostomy diet allows, you can choose to peel the cucumbers to remove any wax or pesticides.

•   Slice the cucumbers thinly for better infusion, ensuring that they can release their flavors into the water effectively.

4. Crush Mint Leaves Gently:

•   Before adding the mint leaves to the water, gently crush them with the back of a spoon or your hands. This helps release the oils and flavors.

5. Use Cold Water:

•   Fill a clean pitcher with cold, filtered water. It's essential to use cold water to avoid releasing any undesirable flavors that can occur with warm water.

6. Combine Ingredients:

•   Add the sliced cucumbers and crushed mint leaves to the cold water in the pitcher.

•   Stir the mixture gently to distribute the flavors evenly.

7. Allow Infusion Time:

• Let the ingredients infuse in the water for at least 1-2 hours. For a more intense flavor, refrigerate the infused water overnight.

8. Strain or Serve As Is:

• Depending on personal preference, you can choose to strain the infused water before serving to remove cucumber and mint particles. Alternatively, leave them in for added visual appeal and a bolder taste.

9. Serve Chilled:

• Serve the cucumber and mint-infused water chilled, either over ice or directly from the refrigerator.

10. Stay Hydrated and Enjoy:

• Incorporate this refreshing beverage into your ileostomy diet to stay hydrated while enjoying a hint of flavor.

• Monitor your body's response to the infused water, especially if you are in the early stages of post-surgery recovery. If any discomfort arises, consult with your healthcare provider.

This Cucumber and Mint Infused Water is not only a delightful and hydrating option but also a great addition to an ostomate's diet, providing a soothing and enjoyable beverage post-surgery. Adjust ingredient quantities and infusion times based on personal preferences and dietary restrictions.

RECIPE 11

YOGURT PARFAIT WITH SOFT BERRIES

When preparing a Yogurt Parfait with Soft Berries for individuals following an ileostomy diet post-surgery, it's essential to consider the specific nutritional needs and digestive sensitivities. Here are detailed preparatory and instructional guidelines:

Ingredients:

1.   **Greek Yogurt:** Opt for plain, unsweetened, and low-fat Greek yogurt. Greek yogurt is rich in protein and can be easier to digest for individuals with an ileostomy.

2.   **Mashed Berries:** Choose soft berries like strawberries, blueberries, or raspberries. Mash them gently to create a juicy and easily digestible texture.

3.   **Optional Add-ins:** Consider adding a touch of honey or a sprinkle of chia seeds for additional nutrients and fiber.

Preparation:

1. Selecting Yogurt:

•   Choose a reputable brand of Greek yogurt with live probiotics. These probiotics can contribute to a healthy gut flora, supporting digestive wellness.

•   Ensure the yogurt is plain and unsweetened to avoid unnecessary added sugars that may cause discomfort.

2. Preparing Mashed Berries:

•   Wash the selected berries thoroughly to remove any contaminants.

•   Gently mash the berries with a fork or potato masher. This not only creates a soft texture but also releases the natural sweetness of the berries.

•   If using strawberries, remove the stems and chop them into small pieces before mashing.

3. Layering the Parfait:

•   Start by spooning a layer of Greek yogurt into a clear glass or bowl.

•   Add a layer of the mashed berries on top of the yogurt.

•   Repeat the process, creating multiple layers of yogurt and berries until the container is filled.

4. Optional Add-ins:

- If desired, drizzle a small amount of honey between the layers for added sweetness. However, be cautious with sweeteners, especially if the individual is sensitive to them.

- Sprinkle a teaspoon of chia seeds between layers to boost the fiber content. Ensure the person has previously tolerated chia seeds well before adding them.

5. Serving and Consumption:

- Serve the yogurt parfait immediately after preparation for the best taste and texture.

- Encourage the individual to eat slowly and savor each bite to aid digestion.

- Monitor for any adverse reactions or discomfort and adjust the recipe accordingly for future servings.

Considerations:

- Consult with a healthcare professional or a dietitian to ensure the chosen ingredients align with the individual's dietary restrictions and preferences.

•   Observe the person's response to the parfait, making note of any foods that may cause discomfort or irritation.

•   Adapt the recipe based on personal preferences and tolerance levels, considering variations like lactose-free yogurt if needed.

This Yogurt Parfait with Soft Berries provides a delicious and nutrient-dense option for individuals following an ileostomy diet, offering a balance of protein, vitamins, and fiber while being gentle on the digestive system.

RECIPE 12

STEAMED ASPARAGUS WITH OLIVE OIL

When preparing Steamed Asparagus with Olive Oil for individuals following an ileostomy diet post-surgery, it's crucial to consider the ease of digestion and the nutritional benefits for abdominal wellness. Here are detailed preparatory and instructional guidelines:

Preparatory Guidelines:

1. Fresh Asparagus Selection:

• Choose fresh, tender asparagus spears. Seek out stiff, erect stalks with firmly closed tips.

• Trim the tough ends by snapping or cutting about 1-2 inches from the bottom. Discard the woody ends.

2. Cleaning and Washing:

• Rinse the asparagus under cold running water to remove any dirt or impurities.

• If desired, you can soak the asparagus in a bowl of cold water for a few minutes and then gently pat it dry.

3. Steam Cooking Equipment:

• Use a steamer basket or an electric steamer for cooking. Steaming helps retain the nutritional value of asparagus.

• Ensure the steaming equipment is clean and sanitized, especially for individuals with post-surgery dietary requirements.

4. Olive Oil Selection:

• Opt for extra-virgin olive oil for its rich flavor and potential health benefits.

• Ensure the olive oil is of high quality and hasn't been heated excessively, as heat can affect its nutritional properties.

5. Portion Control:

• Consider individual dietary restrictions and portion control based on the ostomate's tolerance level.

•   Start with smaller portions initially and gradually increase as tolerance improves.

Instruction Guidelines:

1.   Steaming Process:

•   Place the trimmed asparagus spears in the steamer basket or tray.

•   Steam the asparagus until they are tender yet still slightly crisp. This usually takes 3-5 minutes, depending on the thickness of the spears.

•   Check for doneness by inserting a fork or knife into the thickest part – it should go in easily.

2.   Drizzling with Olive Oil:

•   Once the asparagus is steamed to perfection, transfer them to a serving plate.

•   Drizzle extra-virgin olive oil over the asparagus while they are still warm. The warmth enhances the absorption of flavors and nutrients.

•   Use a brush or spoon to ensure even coating with olive oil.

3.   Seasoning Options:

•   Optionally, add a pinch of salt and pepper for taste. Consider any specific dietary restrictions or preferences while seasoning.

•   Freshly squeezed lemon juice can be added for extra flavor, providing a refreshing touch and additional anti-inflammatory properties.

4.   Serving Suggestions:

•   Serve the steamed asparagus with olive oil as a simple side dish alongside other easily digestible foods suitable for an ileostomy diet.

•   Monitor the individual's response to the dish and adjust ingredients or portions accordingly.

5.   Monitoring Digestive Tolerance:

•   Keep track of how well the individual tolerates the asparagus and olive oil. If well-tolerated, this dish can be incorporated into the post-surgery nutrition plan.

This simple recipe prioritizes ease of digestion, anti-inflammatory properties, and overall abdominal wellness for individuals with an ileostomy, providing a nutritious and flavorful addition to their diet.

RECIPE 13

PUMPKIN AND GINGER SOUP

Preparing a Pumpkin and Ginger Soup for an ileostomy diet involves careful consideration of ingredients and cooking methods to ensure it is gentle on the digestive system post-surgery. Here are the preparatory and instructional guidelines:

Ingredients:

• Pureed Pumpkin

• Fresh Ginger

• Low-sodium Vegetable Broth (optional)

• Salt (to taste, if not using broth)

• Pepper (to taste)

• Olive Oil (optional)

Preparatory Guidelines:

1.   Selecting Ingredients:

•   Choose a fresh, ripe pumpkin for optimal nutritional content.

•   Use fresh ginger, as it adds a delightful flavor and can have potential anti-inflammatory benefits.

•   Opt for low-sodium vegetable broth or prepare your own to control the sodium content.

2.   Cleaning and Peeling:

•   Wash the pumpkin thoroughly before peeling to remove any dirt or contaminants.

•   Peel the pumpkin and remove the seeds. The goal is to have clean, pure pumpkin flesh for easy digestion.

3.   Ginger Preparation:

•   Peel and finely mince or grate the fresh ginger. This ensures that the ginger flavor is evenly distributed in the soup.

Cooking Instructions:

1. Pureeing the Pumpkin:

• Cut the peeled pumpkin into small, uniform pieces for even cooking.

• Steam or boil the pumpkin until it is soft and can be easily pierced with a fork.

• Once cooked, allow the pumpkin to cool slightly before transferring it to a blender or food processor.

2. Blending Process:

• Add the minced or grated ginger to the pumpkin in the blender.

• Blend the mixture until it reaches a smooth, creamy consistency. If the soup is too thick, you can add low-sodium vegetable broth or water gradually until the desired consistency is achieved.

3. Seasoning:

• Add a pinch of salt and pepper to taste. If using low-sodium vegetable broth, adjust the seasoning accordingly.

- Optionally, drizzle a small amount of olive oil for added flavor and healthy fats.

4. Reheating (if needed):

- If the soup has cooled down, gently reheat it on the stovetop. Avoid high heat to preserve the nutritional value of the ingredients.

5. Serving:

- Serve the Pumpkin and Ginger Soup warm.

- Consider garnishing with fresh herbs like cilantro or parsley for an extra burst of flavor.

<u>Important Notes:</u>

- Remember to adapt the recipe to your specific dietary needs and preferences.

- Consult with your healthcare professional or nutritionist to ensure the soup aligns with your post-surgery nutrition plan.

- Monitor your body's response to the soup, and introduce new foods gradually to gauge tolerance.

This Pumpkin and Ginger Soup provides a nourishing option for individuals on an ileostomy diet, promoting abdominal wellness with its gentle and easily digestible ingredients.

RECIPE 14

TENDER TURKEY MEATBALLS

These Tender Turkey Meatballs are designed to provide a protein-packed and easily digestible meal, suitable for individuals with an ileostomy. Ground turkey, combined with breadcrumbs and herbs, creates a flavorful and tender dish that supports post-surgery nutrition.

Preparatory Guidelines:

1. Choose Lean Ground Turkey:

• Opt for lean ground turkey to minimize fat content, making it gentler on the digestive system.

2. High-Quality Breadcrumbs:

• Select high-quality, low-fiber breadcrumbs to enhance the meatball texture without causing digestive distress.

3. Selecting Herbs:

• Use mild and easily digestible herbs such as parsley, chives, or a touch of oregano for added flavor.

[177]

4.   Hydration is Key:

•   Ensure proper hydration during the cooking process. Adequate fluid intake aids digestion and supports overall well-being.

Cooking Instructions:

1.   Preheat the Oven:

•   Preheat the oven to a moderate temperature (around 375°F or 190°C).

2.   Prepare the Turkey Mixture:

•   In a mixing bowl, combine lean ground turkey with the selected breadcrumbs. Add finely chopped herbs for flavor.

3.   Seasoning for Taste:

•   Season the mixture with a pinch of salt and pepper to enhance taste. Be cautious with the salt, as excessive salt intake can lead to dehydration.

4.   Shape into Meatballs: •   With clean hands, gently shape the mixture into evenly sized-meatballs. Keep them small to aid in digestion.

5.   Baking Tray Preparation:

•   Line a baking tray with parchment paper or lightly grease it to prevent sticking.

6.   Evenly Arrange Meatballs:

•   Place the shaped meatballs on the prepared baking tray, ensuring they are evenly spaced for even cooking.

7.   Bake to Perfection:

•   Bake the meatballs in the preheated oven for approximately 20-25 minutes or until they are thoroughly cooked and golden brown. Cooking times may vary, so monitor closely.

8.   Check Internal Temperature:

•   For added safety, use a meat thermometer to ensure the internal temperature reaches at least 165°F (74°C).

9.   Let Them Rest:

• Allow the meatballs to rest for a few minutes after baking. This helps to retain moisture and ensures a tender texture.

Serving Suggestions:

1. Pairing with Suitable Sides:

• Serve the Tender Turkey Meatballs with well-cooked and easily digestible sides such as mashed potatoes or steamed vegetables.

2. Monitor Portion Sizes:

• Control portion sizes to avoid overwhelming the digestive system. Start with a small portion and adjust according to individual tolerance.

3. Chew Thoroughly:

• Encourage thorough chewing to aid in digestion. Smaller, well-chewed bites can help prevent discomfort.

4. Listen to Your Body:

• Pay attention to how your body responds to this meal. If any discomfort or issues arise, adjust ingredients or portion sizes accordingly.

These Tender Turkey Meatballs offer a delicious and nourishing option for individuals on an ileostomy diet. By following these preparatory and instructional guidelines, you can create a meal that supports post-surgery nutrition, ensuring a balance of flavors and easy digestibility.

RECIPE 15

RICE CONGEE WITH SOFT VEGETABLES

When crafting a healing recipe like Rice Congee with Soft Vegetables for individuals undergoing post-surgery nutrition for ileostomy and abdominal wellness, it's crucial to prioritize ingredients and cooking methods that are gentle on the digestive system. Here are detailed preparatory and instructional guidelines:

Ingredients:

1. White Rice:

• Opt for easily digestible white rice. Rinse the rice thoroughly before cooking to remove excess starch, making it gentler on the stomach.

2. Soft Vegetables:

• Choose vegetables that are easy to digest, such as carrots, zucchini, and spinach.

- Wash and chop the vegetables into small, bite-sized pieces to facilitate digestion.

3. Broth:

- Use a mild and low-sodium vegetable or chicken broth to add flavor and enhance the nutritional profile.

- Ensure the broth is strained to eliminate any coarse particles that may irritate the digestive tract.

4. Ginger:

- Incorporate fresh ginger for its anti-inflammatory properties and digestive benefits. Peel and finely chop or grate the ginger before adding it to the congee.

5. Seasonings:

- Keep seasonings simple and mild. Use a pinch of salt or opt for herbs like parsley for added flavor.

Preparation Steps:

1.   Rinse the Rice:

•   Thoroughly rinse the white rice under cold water until the water runs clear. This helps remove excess starch and makes the rice easier to digest.

2.   Cooking the Rice:

•   Use a ratio of 1 cup of rice to 4 cups of broth for a more liquid consistency. Combine the rinsed rice and broth in a pot.

•   Add the chopped ginger for flavor. Bring the mixture to a boil, then reduce the heat to a simmer and cover the pot. Allow it to cook until the rice becomes soft and the congee reaches a porridge-like consistency.

3.   Adding Soft Vegetables:

•   Once the rice is almost cooked, add the chopped soft vegetables to the pot. These vegetables should be easily digestible and complement the gentle nature of the congee.

- Simmer until the vegetables are tender, ensuring they retain their nutritional value.

4. Seasoning:

- Add a pinch of salt or herbs for seasoning. Taste and adjust according to preference, keeping it mild and soothing for the digestive system.

5. Texture Adjustment:

- If needed, adjust the congee's thickness by adding more broth for a lighter consistency or letting it simmer longer for a thicker texture.

6. Serve Warm:

- Allow the congee to cool slightly before serving. Warm foods are often more soothing to the digestive system.

Additional Tips:

- Portion Control:

- Serve small, frequent meals to avoid overwhelming the digestive system. This also helps in better nutrient absorption.

- Hydration:

- Encourage sufficient fluid intake, either through water or clear broths, to prevent dehydration.

- Monitor Reaction:

- Pay attention to the individual's response to the congee. If any discomfort or irritation occurs, consider adjusting the ingredients or consulting a healthcare professional.

Creating a healing recipe like Rice Congee with Soft Vegetables involves a careful balance of gentle ingredients and a cooking process that supports post-surgery nutrition for ileostomy and abdominal wellness. Always tailor the recipe to individual needs and consult with a healthcare professional for personalized dietary advice.

RECIPE 16

GINGER CARROT PUREE

Here are detailed preparatory and instructional guidelines for making Ginger Carrot Puree, a quick and simple healing recipe suitable for an ileostomy diet:

Preparatory Guidelines:

1.   **Choose Fresh Ingredients:** Ensure that you select fresh and high-quality carrots. Look for ones that are firm, brightly colored, and free from blemishes. Fresh ginger with a firm texture and smooth skin is ideal.

2.   **Clean and Peel Carrots:** Wash the carrots thoroughly under running water to remove any dirt. Peel the carrots using a vegetable peeler to eliminate any residual soil and enhance the purity of the puree.

3.   **Cut Carrots into Even Pieces:** Cut the cleaned and peeled carrots into even-sized pieces. This ensures uniform cooking and helps in achieving a smooth consistency when blending.

4. **Prepare Fresh Ginger:** Peel the fresh ginger using the edge of a spoon or a vegetable peeler. Slice or grate the ginger finely. Adjust the amount based on your preference for the intensity of ginger flavor.

Instruction Guidelines:

1. **Cook the Carrots:** Place the prepared carrot pieces in a pot and add enough water to cover them. Upon bringing the water to a boil, lower the heat to a simmer. Cook the carrots until they are tender and can be easily pierced with a fork. Usually, this takes ten to fifteen minutes.

2. **Drain Excess Water:** Once the carrots are cooked, drain any excess water. Retaining a small amount of the cooking liquid can be helpful later in adjusting the consistency of the puree.

3. **Cool the Carrots:** Allow the cooked carrots to cool for a few minutes before transferring them to a blender. This helps avoid steam-related accidents and ensures a safe blending process.

4. **Blend with Fresh Ginger:** Add the cooked carrots and finely sliced or grated ginger to a blender.

Blend until a creamy, smooth consistency is achieved. If the mixture is too thick, you can add a small amount of the reserved cooking liquid to reach your desired texture.

5.   **Check Seasoning:** Taste the puree and adjust the seasoning if needed. You can add a pinch of salt or a dash of pepper for flavor enhancement. Remember that an ileostomy diet may require milder seasoning, so adjust accordingly.

6.   **Serve Warm or Cold:** This Ginger Carrot Puree can be served either warm or cold, depending on your preference. Consider the temperature that feels more soothing and comfortable for your digestive system.

7.   **Storage:** Store any leftover puree in an airtight container in the refrigerator. It can be reheated gently on the stovetop or in the microwave.

8.   **Customization:** Feel free to customize the puree according to your taste preferences. You can experiment with adding a touch of lemon juice, a sprinkle of fresh herbs, or a drizzle of olive oil for extra flavor.

This Ginger Carrot Puree is not only a nourishing addition to an ileostomy diet but also a delightful way to incorporate healing ingredients into your post-surgery nutrition.

Adjust the portion sizes based on your individual dietary needs and consult with your healthcare professional for personalized advice.

RECIPE 17

BANANA ALMOND BUTTER SMOOTHIE

The following guidelines provide a quick and simple recipe along with preparatory instructions to ensure optimal nutrition and abdominal wellness for ostomates.

Preparatory Guidelines:

1.   **Consultation with Healthcare Professionals**: Before incorporating any new recipes into an ileostomy diet, it is crucial to consult with a healthcare professional or a registered dietitian. They can provide personalized advice based on the individual's medical history, nutritional requirements, and recovery status.

2.   **Selecting Ingredients:** Choose fresh and high-quality ingredients for the smoothie. Ensure that the banana is ripe for natural sweetness and easy digestion. Opt for a reputable brand of almond butter, free from

additives, preservatives, or added sugars. Use lactose-free milk to minimize the risk of digestive discomfort.

3. **Washing and Peeling:** Thoroughly wash the banana under running water. Peel the banana and discard the skin. Cleanliness is essential to prevent any potential contaminants that might adversely affect an ostomate's digestive system.

4. **Measuring Ingredients:** Measure the ingredients accurately to maintain portion control and adhere to dietary recommendations. This ensures that the smoothie provides the necessary nutrients without overwhelming the digestive system.

5. **Blender Hygiene:** Clean the blender thoroughly before use to eliminate any residue or potential allergens. Proper hygiene is crucial, especially for individuals with altered digestive systems, to prevent infections or irritations.

6. **Ensuring Almond Butter Quality:** Check the consistency and quality of almond butter. For those who may have difficulty with certain textures, opting for a smooth almond butter might be preferable.

7.   Choosing the Right Lactose-Free Milk: Select a lactose-free milk variant that suits the individual's taste preferences.

This ensures that the smoothie is not only easy on the digestive system but also enjoyable.

Ingredients:

- 1 ripe banana

- 2 tablespoons almond butter

- 1 cup lactose-free milk

Instructions:

1.   Prepare Ingredients: Wash the banana thoroughly under running water. Peel the banana and cut it into smaller chunks for easier blending. Measure two tablespoons of almond butter and ensure the lactose-free milk is ready.

2.   Assemble in Blender: Place the banana chunks, almond butter, and lactose-free milk into the blender. Make sure to add the ingredients in the recommended order to facilitate smooth blending.

3.   Blend Until Smooth: Secure the blender lid and blend the ingredients until smooth. The goal is to achieve a creamy texture for easy consumption and digestion.

4.   Check Consistency: Pause the blender and check the consistency of the smoothie. If it's too thick, add a bit more lactose-free milk and blend again until the desired consistency is reached.

5.   Serve Immediately: Pour the smoothie into a glass and serve immediately. Freshly prepared smoothies offer the best nutritional value and taste.

6.   Optional Additions: For added nutrition, consider incorporating ingredients like chia seeds or a scoop of protein powder. Ensure these additions align with the individual's dietary restrictions and recommendations.

By following these preparatory guidelines and the simple recipe, individuals on an ileostomy diet can enjoy a delicious and nourishing Banana Almond Butter Smoothie while supporting their abdominal wellness during the post-surgery recovery phase.

RECIPE 18

QUINOA AND VEGETABLE STIR-FRY

Preparing a Quinoa and Vegetable Stir-Fry for individuals following an ileostomy diet requires careful attention to ensure the dish is not only delicious but also easy on the digestive system. Here are detailed preparatory and instruction guidelines:

Preparatory Guidelines:

1. Choose High-Quality Ingredients:

• Select fresh, high-quality quinoa to maximize nutritional benefits.

• Opt for organic vegetables to minimize exposure to pesticides and additives.

2. Rinse Quinoa Thoroughly:

• Rinse quinoa under cold water to remove the bitter outer coating called saponin.

• Use a fine-mesh strainer to ensure thorough cleaning.

3. Vegetable Preparation:

• Wash and chop vegetables into bite-sized pieces.

• Consider steaming or blanching veggies slightly for easier digestion.

4. Cooking Utensils:

• Use non-stick pans to minimize the need for excessive oil.

• Use a spatula to gently stir the ingredients without irritating them.

5. Timing Consideration:

• Plan your cooking time to allow for relaxed preparation without rushing.

• Consider preparing ingredients in advance for a quicker assembly.

Instruction Guidelines:

1. Cooking Quinoa:

a. Water Ratio: Use a 1:2 ratio of quinoa to water for optimal fluffiness. b. Boiling: Bring water to a boil, add quinoa, and simmer until water is absorbed. c. Fluffing: Let it sit for a few minutes, then fluff with a fork.

2. Soft Stir-Frying Vegetables:

a. Minimal Oil: Use a small amount of olive oil or a light oil of your choice. b. Medium Heat: Heat the pan to medium to avoid excessive browning. c. Add Vegetables Gradually: Start with carrots, followed by bell peppers, and lastly zucchini for even cooking. d. Seasoning: Add salt and pepper sparingly for flavor without overwhelming the digestive system.

3. Combining Quinoa and Vegetables:

a. Gentle Mixing: Combine the cooked quinoa with stir-fried vegetables gently to avoid breaking down the grains. b. Adjust Seasoning: Taste and adjust seasoning if needed, keeping in mind the sensitivity of the digestive system.

4. Serving Suggestions:

a. Portion Control: Serve moderate portions to prevent overeating. b. Chewing Thoroughly: Encourage individuals to chew slowly and thoroughly to aid digestion.

5. Accompaniments:

• Consider serving with a light, homemade sauce like a lemon vinaigrette for added flavor without overwhelming the dish.

6. Hydration:

• Encourage consuming water before and after the meal to aid digestion.

7. Observation:

• Observe for any adverse reactions or discomfort during and after consumption.

This Quinoa and Vegetable Stir-Fry provides a well-balanced, nutrient-dense option for individuals on an ileostomy diet, focusing on both flavor and digestive ease. Adjust ingredient quantities and cooking methods based on individual preferences and tolerances.

RECIPE 19

SALMON AND SWEET POTATO MASH

Preparing a healing and nutritious meal like Salmon and Sweet Potato Mash for individuals following an ileostomy diet requires careful consideration. **Here are detailed preparatory and instructional guidelines:**

1. Salmon Selection:

• Opt for fresh or frozen wild-caught salmon, as it is a rich source of omega-3 fatty acids. Ensure that the salmon is properly cleaned, deboned, and skinless.

2. Sweet Potato Preparation:

• Choose fresh sweet potatoes, preferably organic. Peel and dice them into uniform chunks for even cooking.

- Sweet potatoes are high in fiber and vitamins, providing a good source of complex carbohydrates. Their natural sweetness adds flavor without the need for added sugars.

3. Baking the Salmon:

- Preheat the oven to 375°F (190°C).

- Season the salmon fillet with a pinch of salt, pepper, and a dash of olive oil for moisture.

- Place the seasoned salmon on a baking sheet lined with parchment paper to prevent sticking.

- Bake for approximately 15-20 minutes or until the salmon is cooked through and flakes easily with a fork.

4. Cooking Sweet Potatoes:

- Boil the diced sweet potatoes until they are tender but not mushy. This usually takes about 15-20 minutes, depending on the size of the potato chunks.

- Drain the sweet potatoes and let them cool slightly before mashing.

5. Mashing Sweet Potatoes:

- Mash the cooked sweet potatoes using a potato masher or fork. Use a food processor or blender for a smoother consistency.

- Add a touch of unsalted butter or olive oil for added flavor and moisture.

- Season with salt and pepper to taste.

6. Assembling the Dish:

- Once the salmon is baked and the sweet potatoes are mashed, place a serving of the mashed sweet potatoes on a plate.

- Top the sweet potatoes with the baked salmon fillet.

- Garnish with fresh herbs like parsley or dill for additional flavor and a pop of color.

7. Serving Suggestions:

- Serve the Salmon and Sweet Potato Mash warm to enhance the flavors.

- Consider adding a side of steamed vegetables or a light salad for added vitamins and minerals.

8. Portion Control:

•   Pay attention to portion sizes, as overeating can be challenging for individuals with an ileostomy. Smaller, frequent meals may be better tolerated.

9. Hydration:

•   Accompany the meal with plenty of water to stay well-hydrated, which is essential for digestion and overall well-being.

10. Consultation with Healthcare Provider:

•   Before introducing new foods into the ileostomy diet, it's advisable to consult with a healthcare provider or a registered dietitian to ensure compatibility with individual health conditions.

This Salmon and Sweet Potato Mash provides a balanced mix of nutrients, offering a gentle and nourishing option for individuals recovering from surgery and managing an ileostomy.

RECIPE 20

CAULIFLOWER RICE BOWL WITH SOFT CHICKEN

Preparing a Cauliflower Rice Bowl with Soft Chicken is a great choice for individuals following an ileostomy diet. This recipe provides a low-carb, easy-to-digest option that is gentle on the digestive system post-surgery. Here are detailed preparatory and instruction guidelines:

Ingredients:

1. **Cauliflower Rice:**

- 1 medium-sized cauliflower head

- Olive oil

- Salt and pepper to taste

2. **Soft Chicken:**

- 2 boneless, skinless chicken breasts

- Olive oil

- Salt and pepper to taste

Instructions:

1. Preparing Cauliflower Rice:

• Wash the cauliflower head thoroughly and cut it into smaller florets.

• Using a food processor, pulse the cauliflower florets until they reach a rice-like consistency. Be cautious not to over-process, as you want a slightly coarse texture.

• In a large skillet, heat a tablespoon of olive oil over medium heat.

• Add the cauliflower rice to the skillet and sauté for 5-7 minutes, stirring occasionally. Season with salt and pepper to taste.

• Cook until the cauliflower rice is tender but not mushy. Set aside.

2. Cooking Soft Chicken:

• Season the chicken breasts with salt and pepper on both sides.

- In a separate skillet, heat a tablespoon of olive oil over medium-high heat.

- Add the seasoned chicken breasts to the skillet and cook for about 4-5 minutes on each side or until fully cooked.

- Once cooked, remove the chicken from the skillet and let it rest for a few minutes.

- Shred the chicken using two forks or your hands, creating soft and easily digestible strands.

3. Putting the Cauliflower Rice Bowl Together:

- Divide the cauliflower rice among serving bowls.

- Top the cauliflower rice with the shredded chicken.

- Optionally, you can add additional toppings such as chopped fresh herbs, a squeeze of lemon juice, or a drizzle of olive oil for extra flavor.

- Mix gently to combine the ingredients evenly.

4. Serving and Storage:

- Serve the Cauliflower Rice Bowl warm.

- This dish can be stored in airtight containers in the refrigerator for up to 2-3 days. Reheat gently in the microwave before serving.

5. Considerations for Ileostomy Diet:

- Ensure that the cauliflower is cooked to a soft texture to ease digestion.

- Choose lean cuts of chicken to minimize fat content.

- Portion control is important, and individuals should monitor their tolerance to different foods.

This Cauliflower Rice Bowl with Soft Chicken provides a nutritious, easy-to-digest meal for individuals following an ileostomy diet. It's important to listen to your body's response to different foods and make adjustments based on your tolerance and preferences.

RECIPE 21

MANGO BANANA YOGURT PARFAIT

Preparatory and Instruction Guidelines for Mango Banana Yogurt Parfait in the context of an Ileostomy Diet:

1. Clean and Sanitize:

• Wash hands thoroughly with soap and water before handling any ingredients.

• Ensure all utensils, cutting boards, and surfaces are clean and sanitized to prevent any risk of contamination, especially considering post-surgery dietary needs.

2. Choose Ripe Ingredients:

• Select ripe mangoes and bananas for the best flavor and nutrient content.

•   Ripe fruits are usually softer and easier to digest, making them suitable for individuals following an ileostomy diet.

3. Prepare the Mango:

•   Peel the mango and carefully cut it into small, bite-sized cubes.

•   Remove the pit, as it may be challenging for some individuals with an ileostomy to digest.

4. Slice the Banana:

•   Peel the banana and slice it into thin rounds.

•   Opt for well-ripened bananas for a sweeter taste and smoother digestion.

5. Choose Lactose-Free Yogurt:

•   Ensure the yogurt chosen is lactose-free to accommodate potential digestive sensitivities.

•   Greek yogurt or other thick varieties may provide additional protein and creaminess.

6. Layering:

- Begin by placing a spoonful of lactose-free yogurt at the bottom of a clean, clear glass or bowl.

- Add a layer of diced mango on top of the yogurt.

- Follow with a layer of banana slices.

- Repeat the layering process until the glass or bowl is filled, creating a visually appealing parfait.

7. Portion Control:

- Keep portion sizes moderate to prevent overwhelming the digestive system.

- Smaller, more frequent meals may be better tolerated for individuals with an ileostomy.

8. Serve Chilled:

- For added comfort, refrigerate the parfait before serving.

- A chilled parfait can be soothing and refreshing, especially during the recovery period after surgery.

9. Variations:

- Consider incorporating other easily digestible fruits like berries or kiwi for additional nutritional variety.

- Experiment with different lactose-free yogurt flavors to suit individual preferences.

10. Hydration:

- Remember to stay well-hydrated throughout the day, as hydration is crucial for optimal digestion and overall health.

- Consider sipping water or a clear beverage alongside the parfait.

11. Listen to Your Body:

- Pay attention to how your body responds to the parfait. Everyone's tolerance level may vary, so adjust the ingredients or portion sizes accordingly.

This Mango Banana Yogurt Parfait offers a delightful combination of flavors, vitamins, and gentle textures, making it a suitable choice for individuals on an ileostomy diet seeking post-surgery nutrition for abdominal wellness. Adjustments can be made based on personal preferences and specific dietary needs.

RECIPE 22

LEMON HERB BAKED COD

The Lemon Herb Baked Cod is an excellent choice, offering a light and flavorful option rich in essential nutrients to support overall abdominal wellness. Here are detailed preparatory and instructional guidelines for this healing recipe:

Preparation:

1.   Choose Fresh Cod Fillets:

•   Select fresh, high-quality cod fillets from a reputable source. Freshness is key to ensuring optimal nutritional value and taste.

2.   Gentle Thawing:

• If using frozen cod, thaw it gradually in the refrigerator to maintain its texture and prevent loss of moisture.

3. Gather Ingredients:

• Ensure you have all the necessary ingredients on hand:

• Cod fillets

• Fresh lemons

• Assorted herbs (such as parsley, dill, or thyme)

• Olive oil

• Salt and pepper

4. Preheat Oven:

• Preheat your oven to a moderate temperature, usually around 375°F (190°C), ensuring even cooking without compromising the delicate nature of the fish.

5. Prepare a Baking Dish:

- Choose a baking dish that comfortably accommodates the cod fillets without overcrowding. Lightly grease the dish to prevent sticking.

Instruction:

1.   Season the Cod:

- Place the cod fillets in the prepared baking dish. Squeeze fresh lemon juice over the fillets, ensuring even coverage.

- Sprinkle a mixture of finely chopped herbs over the cod. Common choices include parsley, dill, or thyme, but feel free to tailor it to personal preferences.

- Drizzle a touch of olive oil over the fillets, providing a healthy source of fats that aids in nutrient absorption.

2.   Add Salt and Pepper:

- Season the cod with a pinch of salt and pepper. Use these sparingly, as the goal is to enhance flavors without overwhelming the dish or causing digestive discomfort.

3.   Gentle Mixing:

• Gently toss the cod fillets in the seasoning, ensuring that each piece is coated evenly. Be careful not to break or damage the delicate fish.

4. Bake to Perfection:

• Place the baking dish in the preheated oven and bake for approximately 15-20 minutes or until the cod is cooked through and flakes easily with a fork.

• Keep an eye on the cooking process to prevent overcooking, as this could affect the tenderness of the cod.

5. Serve with Care:

• Once baked, carefully transfer the cod fillets to a serving plate. Ensure that the fillets remain intact to preserve both their presentation and texture.

6. Accompaniments:

• Consider serving the Lemon Herb Baked Cod with sides that are gentle on the digestive system, such as steamed vegetables or a light salad. These add nutritional value without adding unnecessary strain.

7. Portion Control:

- Be mindful of portion sizes, allowing for a balanced meal that supports abdominal wellness without overwhelming the digestive system.

This Lemon Herb Baked Cod recipe not only provides essential nutrients but also introduces flavors that are comforting and enjoyable, making it a valuable addition to the ileostomy diet post-surgery. Adjust the seasonings and cooking times according to personal preferences and dietary needs, always prioritizing the gentle nature of the meal for optimal healing.

RECIPE 23
SPINACH AND FETA OMELETTE

Preparing a Spinach and Feta Omelette for an ileostomy diet requires careful consideration of ingredients and cooking methods to ensure it is gentle on the digestive system and promotes abdominal wellness post-surgery. Here are detailed preparatory and instructional guidelines:

Preparatory Guidelines:

1.   Choose Fresh Ingredients:

•   Opt for fresh eggs, preferably organic, to ensure a high-quality protein source.

•   Select fresh spinach, as it is rich in vitamins and minerals. Ensure it is thoroughly washed to remove any debris.

2.   Crumbled Feta Cheese:

- Use a high-quality, low-sodium feta cheese. It adds flavor without overwhelming the dish with excessive salt, which may be sensitive for individuals with an ileostomy.

3. Whisking Eggs:

- Crack the eggs into a clean bowl. Make sure there are no remaining pieces of shell.

- Whisk the eggs thoroughly to create a uniform mixture. This aids in achieving a light and fluffy texture in the omelet.

4. Sautéing Spinach:

- Heat a non-stick skillet over medium heat. Add a small amount of olive oil or a suitable oil of your choice.

- Sauté the spinach until it wilts. This not only enhances the flavor but also makes it easier to digest.

Instructional Guidelines:

1. Prepare the Eggs:

- In a mixing bowl, whisk the eggs until the yolks and whites are well combined. This step is crucial to achieving a uniform texture in the omelet.

2. Sauté the Spinach:

- In a non-stick skillet, add a small amount of oil over medium heat.

- Add the sautéed spinach to the whisked eggs. This adds a nutrient boost and a gentle, easy-to-digest vegetable component to the dish.

3. Cooking the Omelette:

- Pour the egg and spinach mixture into the skillet.

- Allow the mixture to set around the edges before gently lifting the sides with a spatula, allowing the uncooked egg to flow underneath.

- Once the majority of the egg is set, sprinkle crumbled feta cheese evenly over one-half of the omelet.

4. Folding the Omelette:

- Carefully fold the other half of the omelet over the side with the feta cheese, creating a half-moon shape.

- Press down gently with the spatula to ensure the cheese melts and binds the omelet together.

5. Serve Warm:

- Transfer the omelet to a plate and allow it to cool slightly before serving.

- For added flavor, you can sprinkle a small amount of fresh herbs, such as chives or parsley, on top.

6. Accompaniments:

- Consider serving the omelet with well-cooked, easy-to-digest grains like white rice or quinoa to provide additional nutrients and energy.

7. Portion Control:

- Keep portions moderate to avoid overwhelming the digestive system. Listen to your body and adjust portion sizes based on individual comfort.

By following these preparatory and instructional guidelines, you can create a delicious and nutritious

Spinach and Feta Omelette suitable for individuals on an ileostomy diet, promoting post-surgery nutrition and abdominal wellness.

APPRECIATION

Dear Beloved Customers,

I am overwhelmed with gratitude as I reflect upon the journey that led to the creation of the "***ILEOSTOMY DIET: POST-SURGERY NUTRITION FOR OSTOMATE ABDOMINAL WELLNESS***." This project has been a labor of love, a testament to the strength that arises from adversity, and a celebration of the human spirit's ability to overcome challenges.

To the Almighty, I extend my deepest appreciation for the wisdom, inspiration, and guidance that made this endeavor possible. It is with profound gratitude that I acknowledge your divine presence in every step of this creative process. Your grace has fueled the pages of this cookbook, providing a source of hope and wellness for those navigating the challenging path of post-surgery recovery.

To my cherished customers, thank you for entrusting me with a small part of your journey toward digestive wellness. Crafting this cookbook was a heartfelt effort to support and empower individuals adapting to life with an ileostomy. Your faith in my work fuels my passion, and it is my sincerest hope that these recipes, meal ideas, and preparation tips bring comfort, joy, and nourishment to your daily life.

I humbly urges you to share your thoughts and experiences by providing feedback, rating, and reviewing this book "Ileostomy Diet: Post-Surgery Nutrition For Ostomate Abdominal Wellness." Your valuable insights will guide me in refining and enhancing future editions, ensuring that I continue to meet your needs and expectations. Your voices matter, and your input is a beacon of light that steers this ship towards even greater shores.

As you delve into the world of low-fiber, low-residue ileostomy recovery, I urge you to not only find solace within the pages of this cookbook but also to share the treasure you've discovered with others. Recommend and spread the word to friends, family, and loved ones who may benefit from the wealth of knowledge within these pages. Together, let us create a ripple effect of support and healthy living, extending the reach of this cookbook's impact far and wide.

Thank you, once again, for being an integral part of this journey. May the "Ileostomy Diet - Post-Surgery Nutrition for Ostomate Abdominal Wellness" be a source of comfort, inspiration, and resilience for all who embark on the path of digestive wellness.

With heartfelt appreciation,

[Dr. Ruben Berry]

Made in the USA
Columbia, SC
01 May 2025

57423643R10124